COMMITTEE TO STUDY THE HEALTH-RELATED EFFECTS
OF CANNABIS AND ITS DERIVATIVES

Arnold S. Relman, Chairman
Editor
The New England Journal of Medicine

Konrad E. Bloch
Professor
Department of Chemistry
Harvard University

Barton Childs
Professor of Pediatrics
  and Biology
The Johns Hopkins University
  School of Medicine

Michael I. Cohen
Chairman and Professor
Department of Pediatrics
Albert Einstein College
  of Medicine
Montefiore Hospital and
  Medical Center

P. B. Dews
Professor of Psychiatry
  and Psychobiology
Laboratory of Psychobiology
Harvard Medical School

Edward F. Domino
Professor
Department of Pharmacology
University of Michigan

Robert B. Edgerton
Professor
Departments of Psychiatry
  and Anthropology
University of California,
  Los Angeles

Daniel D. Federman
Dean for Students and Alumni
Harvard Medical School

Irwin Feinberg
Professor of Psychiatry
University of California,
  San Francisco and
Veterans Administration Medical
  Center, San Francisco

Alfred P. Fishman
Professor of Medicine
Director
Cardiovascular Pulmonary Division
Hospital of the University
  of Pennsylvania

Beatrix Hamburg
Associate Professor of Psychiatry
Department of Psychiatry and
  Department of Social Medicine
  and Health Policy
Harvard Medical School

H. Carl Haywood
Professor of Psychology
  and Neurology
Director
The John F. Kennedy Center
  for Research on Education
  and Human Development
Vanderbilt University

Reese T. Jones
Professor of Psychiatry
Langley Porter Psychiatric
  Institute
University of California,
  San Francisco

Harold Kalant
Professor
Department of Pharmacology
University of Toronto

Denise Kandel
Professor of Public Health
Department of Psychiatry
Columbia University and
New York State Psychiatric
   Institute

Barbara M. Korsch
Professor of Pediatrics
   and Head
Division of General Pediatrics
Children's Hospital of
   Los Angeles
University of Southern California
   School of Medicine

Robert Y. Moore
Professor and Chairman
Department of Neurology
State University of New York
   at Stony Brook

Robert F. Murray, Jr.
Professor of Pediatrics,
   Medicine and Oncology
Chief, Division of Medical Genetics
Department of Pediatrics and Child
   Health
College of Medicine
Howard University

Norton Nelson
Professor of Environmental
   Medicine
New York University
   Medical Center

Charles P. O'Brien
Professor of Psychiatry
University of Pennsylvania
   School of Medicine and
Philadelphia Veterans Adminis-
   tration Medical Center

Sheldon J. Segal
Director
Population Sciences Division
Rockefeller Foundation

Paul D. Stolley
Professor
Department of Medicine
University of Pennsylvania
   School of Medicine

iv

Marijuana and Health

Report of a Study
by a Committee of the
INSTITUTE OF MEDICINE
Division of Health Sciences Policy

NATIONAL ACADEMY PRESS
Washington, D.C.   1982

NOTICE The project that is the subject of this report was approved by the Governing Board of the National Research Council, whose members are drawn from the Councils of the National Academy of Sciences, the National Academy of Engineering, and the Institute of Medicine. The members of the committee responsible for the report were chosen for their special competences and with regard for appropriate balance.

This report has been reviewed by a group other than the authors according to procedures approved by a Report Review Committee consisting of members of the National Academy of Sciences, the National Academy of Engineering, and the Institute of Medicine.

The Institute of Medicine was chartered in 1970 by the National Academy of Sciences to enlist distinguished members of the appropriate professions in the examination of policy matters pertaining to the health of the public. In this, the Institute acts under both the Academy's 1863 Congressional charter responsibility to be an advisor to the federal government, and its own initiative in identifying issues of medical care, research, and education.

This study was supported by the National Institutes of Health, Contract No. NO1-OD-0-2114.

International Standard Book Number 0-309-03236-9

Library of Congress Catalog Card Number 81-86534

Available from:

NATIONAL ACADEMY PRESS
2101 Constitution Ave., N.W.
Washington, D.C. 20418

Printed in the United States of America

INSTITUTE OF MEDICINE
Frederick C. Robbins
President

Study Staff

Enriqueta C. Bond, Director, Division of Health Sciences Policy

Linda S. Dujack, Study Director

Kathryn G. King, Research Associate

Caren M. Carney, Research Associate

Allyn M. Mortimer, Research Assistant

Roszel S. Thomsen II, Research Assistant

Linda A. DePugh, Administrative Secretary

Constance V. Shuck, Administrative Secretary

With the collaboration of the Director of the Division of Mental Health and Behavioral Medicine, Fredric Solomon, and the assistance of Institute of Medicine staff members Barbara Filner, Barbara Mandula, and Robert Field.

Consultants

Henry D. Abraham, Harvard University

Richard E. Belleville, Private Consultant

Kevin Fehr, Addiction Research Foundation

Herbert Moskowitz, Southern California Research Institute

Wendy Nelson, University of Pennsylvania

Oakley S. Ray, Veterans Administration Medical Center

Brian L. Strom, University of Pennsylvania

Study of the Health-Related Effects of
Cannabis and Its Derivatives

PANELS

Cardiovascular and Respiratory Issues

Alfred P. Fishman*, Chairman

Brian F. Hoffman
Professor and Chairman
Department of Pharmacology
Columbia University College
  of Physicians and Surgeons

Gerard M. Turino
Professor of Medicine
Department of Medicine
Columbia University College
  of Physicians and Surgeons

Jerome I. Kleinerman
Chairman
Department of Pathology
Mount Sinai School of Medicine

Neurobiological Issues

Irwin Feinberg*, Chairman

Edward F. Domino*

H. Craig Heller
Associate Professor of Biology
Department of Biological Sciences
Stanford University

Reese T. Jones*

Harold Kalant*

Irwin H. Krakoff
Director
Vermont Regional Cancer Center

A. Edward Maumenee
Professor of Ophthalmology
Wilmer Institute
Johns Hopkins Hospital

Robert Moore*

Charles P. O'Brien*

_____

*Committee member.

Behavioral, Psychosocial, and Epidemiologic Issues

Charles P. O'Brien* and H. Carl Haywood*, Co-Chairmen

Michael I. Cohen*

Robert B. Edgerton*

Beatrix Hamburg*

Reese T. Jones*

Denise Kandel*

Barbara M. Korsch*

Paul D. Stolley*

Reproductive and Fetal Issues

Daniel D. Federman*, Chairman

F. Clarke Fraser
Director of Medical Genetics
Montreal Children's Hospital

Norton Nelson*

Sheldon Segal*

Genetic, Oncogenic, and Cytogenetic Issues

Barton Childs*, Chairman

Arthur D. Bloom
Professor of Pediatrics and of
  Human Genetics and Development
Director, Clinical Genetics
Columbia University College
  of Physicians and Surgeons

Robert F. Murray, Jr.*

Norton Nelson*

Dietrich Hoffmann
Associate Director
Naylor Dana Institute for
  Disease Prevention

Cell Biology, Pharmacology, and Immunological Issues

P. B. Dews*, Chairman

Konrad E. Bloch*

Reese T. Jones*

Louis Lemberger
Director of Clinical
  Pharmacology
Lilly Laboratory for
  Clinical Research

Peter H. Schur
Professor of Medicine
Harvard University
Brigham and Women's Hospital

_____
*Committee member.

ACKNOWLEDGMENTS

Many persons outside the Institute of Medicine provided helpful
suggestions, timely observations, and data bearing on the complex
scientific, clinical, and societal issues that were being explored by
the committee and staff. We wish especially to express our gratitude
for contributions made by Monique Braude, Jacqueline Ludford, Robert
Petersen, William Pollin, and Marvin Snyder of the National Institute
on Drug Abuse; Edward Tocus and Stuart Nightingale of the Food and
Drug Administration; the Interagency Committee to Monitor the
Marijuana Study; Carl Leventhal of the National Institutes of Health
and the chairman of the Interagency Committee; and Joseph Perpich of
the National Institutes of Health, our project officer.
    We wish also to acknowledge the many scientists and others who
responded to specific requests to review informally a portion of the
draft report and those who, in general, gave their active assistance
and collaboration:

- C. Wayne Bardin, Population Council
- Neal Benowitz, Langley Porter Psychiatric Institute
- Albert Carlin, University of Washington
- Sidney Cohen, Alcohol Research Center
- Ellen Dempsey, McGill University
- Everett Ellinwood, Duke University Medical Center
- Keith Green, Medical College of Georgia
- Daniel Hoth, National Cancer Institute
- Lloyd Johnston, Institute for Social Research
- Louise Lev, National Cancer Institute
- Markku Linnoila, National Institute of Mental Health
- Oriana Kalant and the Documentation Center of the Addiction
  Research Foundation
- Edward Khantzian, Cambridge Hospital
- Kaye Kilburn, University of Southern California School of
  Medicine
- Warren Levinson, University of California, San Francisco
- Raphael Mechoulam, School of Pharmacy, The Hebrew
  University, Israel
- John Merritt, University of North Carolina

- Akira Morishima, College of Physicians and Surgeons, Columbia University
- Al Munson, Medical College of Virginia
- Gabriel Nahas, College of Physicians and Surgeons, Columbia University
- William Paton, University of Oxford
- Bruce Petersen, Lilly Laboratory for Clinical Research
- Steven Podas, the Mount Sinai Medical Center
- Lee Robins, Washington University Medical School
- Harris Rosenkrantz, EG&G Mason Research Institute
- Donald Tashkin, University of California, Los Angeles
- David Taylor, Centers for Disease Control
- Carlton Turner, Senior Policy Adviser for Drug Policy, Office of Policy Development
- Arthur Zimmerman, University of Toronto

PREFACE

This report is the work of the many people identified in the preceding pages, and to all of them I am very grateful. I particularly wish to thank my distinguished colleagues on the study committee, upon whose expert knowledge and critical judgment this report rests. They responded conscientiously to all the demands placed on them, and they did so with a promptness and grace that made my task easy.

No study of this kind can be carried out without the help of a skilled staff. We were fortunate to have had the assistance of a devoted and highly capable staff team led by Enriqueta C. Bond and Linda S. Dujack. They coordinated the efforts of the committee, the panel, the consultants, and the Institute of Medicine staff, and they played the key role in keeping everything on schedule. Moreover, they carried out this formidable task with tact and common sense. On behalf of the committee, I wish publicly to acknowledge our indebtedness to the IOM staff, and I also wish to express my personal thanks to Drs. Bond and Dujack for their unfailing support and cooperation.

Finally, I wish to acknowledge my appreciation of the editorial assistance of Wallace K. Waterfall, whose expert touch is evident throughout this document. Our aim was to write a report in "a clear and incisive form for the general public." Any success that we may have achieved is due in no small measure to his efforts.

Arnold S. Relman, M.D.
Chairman

CONTENTS

Marijuana and Health

SUMMARY

The Institute of Medicine (IOM) of the National Academy of Sciences has conducted a 15-month study of the health-related effects of marijuana, at the request of the Secretary of Health and Human Services and the Director of the National Institutes of Health. The IOM appointed a 22-member committee to:

* analyze existing scientific evidence bearing on the possible hazards to the health and safety of users of marijuana;
* analyze data concerning the possible therapeutic value and health benefits of marijuana;
* assess federal research programs in marijuana;
* identify promising new research directions, and make suggestions to improve the quality and usefulness of future research; and
* draw conclusions from this review that would accurately assess the limits of present knowledge and thereby provide a factual, scientific basis for the development of future government policy.

This assessment of knowledge of the health-related effects of marijuana is important and timely because marijuana is now the most widely used of all the illicit drugs available in the United States. In 1979, more than 50 million persons had tried it at least once. There has been a steep rise in its use during the past decade, particularly among adolescents and young adults, although there has been a leveling-off in its overall use among high school seniors in the past 2 or 3 years and a small decline in the percentage of seniors who use it frequently. Although substantially more high school students have used alcohol than have ever used marijuana, more high school seniors use marijuana on a daily or near-daily basis (9 percent) than alcohol (6 percent). Much of the heavy use of marijuana, unlike alcohol, takes place in school, where effects on behavior, cognition, and psychomotor performance can be particularly disturbing. Unlike alcohol, which is rapidly metabolized and eliminated from the body, the psychoactive components of marijuana persist in the body for a long time. Similar to alcohol, continued use of marijuana may cause tolerance and dependence. For all these reasons, it is imperative that we have reliable and detailed information about the effects of marijuana use on health, both in the long and short term.

What, then, did we learn from our review of the published scientific literature? Numerous acute effects have been described in animals, in isolated cells and tissues, and in studies of human volunteers; clinical and epidemiological observations also have been reported. This information is briefly summarized in the following paragraphs.

EFFECTS ON THE NERVOUS SYSTEM AND ON BEHAVIOR

We can say with confidence that marijuana produces acute effects on the brain, including chemical and electrophysiological changes. Its most clearly established acute effects are on mental functions and behavior. With a severity directly related to dose, marijuana impairs motor coordination and affects tracking ability and sensory and perceptual functions important for safe driving and the operation of other machines; it also impairs short-term memory and slows learning. Other acute effects include feelings of euphoria and other mood changes, but there also are disturbing mental phenomena, such as brief periods of anxiety, confusion, or psychosis.

There is not yet any conclusive evidence as to whether prolonged use of marijuana causes permanent changes in the nervous system or sustained impairment of brain function and behavior in human beings. In a few unconfirmed studies in experimental animals, impairment of learning and changes in electrical brain-wave recordings have been observed several months after the cessation of chronic administration of marijuana. In the judgment of the committee, widely cited studies purporting to demonstrate that marijuana affects the gross and microscopic structure of the human or monkey brain are not convincing; much more work is needed to settle this important point.

Chronic relatively heavy use of marijuana is associated with behavioral dysfunction and mental disorders in human beings, but available evidence does not establish if marijuana use under these circumstances is a cause or a result of the mental condition. There are similar problems in interpreting the evidence linking the use of marijuana to subsequent use of other illicit drugs, such as heroin or cocaine. Association does not prove a causal relation, and the use of marijuana may merely be symptomatic of an underlying disposition to use psychoactive drugs rather than a "stepping stone" to involvement with more dangerous substances. It is also difficult to sort out the relationship between use of marijuana and the complex symptoms known as the amotivational syndrome. Self-selection and effects of the drug are probably both contributing to the motivational problems seen in some chronic users of marijuana.

Thus, the long-term effects of marijuana on the human brain and on human behavior remain to be defined. Although we have no convincing evidence thus far of any effects persisting in human beings after cessation of drug use, there may well be subtle but important physical and psychological consequences that have not been recognized.

EFFECTS ON THE CARDIOVASCULAR AND RESPIRATORY SYSTEMS

There is good evidence that the smoking of marijuana usually causes acute changes in the heart and circulation that are characteristic of stress, but there is no evidence to indicate that a permanently deleterious effect on the normal cardiovascular system occurs. There is good evidence to show that marijuana increases the work of the heart, usually by raising heart rate and, in some persons, by raising blood pressure. This rise in workload poses a threat to patients with hypertension, cerebrovascular disease, and coronary atherosclerosis.

Acute exposure to marijuana smoke generally elicits bronchodilation; chronic heavy smoking of marijuana causes inflammation and pre-neoplastic changes in the airways, similar to those produced by smoking of tobacco. Marijuana smoke is a complex mixture that not only has many chemical components (including carbon monoxide and "tar") and biological effects similar to those of tobacco smoke, but also some unique ingredients. This suggests the strong possibility that prolonged heavy smoking of marijuana, like tobacco, will lead to cancer of the respiratory tract and to serious impairment of lung function. Although there is evidence of impaired lung function in chronic smokers, no direct confirmation of the likelihood of cancer has yet been provided, possibly because marijuana has been widely smoked in this country for only about 20 years, and data have not been collected systematically in other countries with a much longer history of heavy marijuana use.

EFFECTS ON THE REPRODUCTIVE SYSTEM AND ON CHROMOSOMES

Although studies in animals have shown that Δ-9-THC (the major psychoactive constituent of marijuana) lowers the concentration in blood serum of pituitary hormones (gonadotropins) that control reproductive functions, it is not known if there is a direct effect on reproductive tissues. Delta-9-THC appears to have a modest reversible suppressive effect on sperm production in men, but there is no proof that it has a deleterious effect on male fertility. Effects on human female hormonal function have been reported, but the evidence is not convincing. However, there is convincing evidence that marijuana interferes with ovulation in female monkeys. No satisfactory studies of the relation between use of marijuana and female fertility and child-bearing have been carried out. Although Δ-9-THC is known to cross the placenta readily and to cause birth defects when administered in large doses to experimental animals, no adequate clinical studies have been carried out to determine if marijuana use can harm the human fetus. There is no conclusive evidence of teratogenicity in human offspring, but a slowly developing or low-level effect might be undetected by the studies done so far. The effects of marijuana on reproductive function and on the fetus are unclear; they may prove to be negligible, but further research to establish or rule out such effects would be of great importance.

Extracts from marijuana smoke particulates ("tar") have been found to produce dose-related mutations in bacteria; however, Δ-9-THC, by itself, is not mutagenic. Marijuana and Δ-9-THC do not appear to break chromosomes, but marijuana may affect chromosome segregation during cell division, resulting in an abnormal number of chromosomes in daughter cells. Although these results are of concern, their clinical significance is unknown.

THE IMMUNE SYSTEM

Similar limitations exist in our understanding of the effects of marijuana on other body systems. For example, some studies of the immune system demonstrate a mild, immunosuppressant effect on human beings, but other studies show no effect.

THERAPEUTIC POTENTIAL

The committee also has examined the evidence on the therapeutic effects of marijuana in a variety of medical disorders. Preliminary studies suggest that marijuana and its derivatives or analogues might be useful in the treatment of the raised intraocular pressure of glaucoma, in the control of the severe nausea and vomiting caused by cancer chemotherapy, and in the treatment of asthma. There also is some preliminary evidence that a marijuana constituent (cannabidiol) might be helpful in the treatment of certain types of epileptic seizures, as well as for spastic disorders and other nervous system diseases. But, in these and all other conditions, much more work is needed. Because marijuana and Δ-9-THC often produce troublesome psychotropic or cardiovascular side-effects that limit their therapeutic usefulness, particularly in older patients, the greatest therapeutic potential probably lies in the use of synthetic analogues of marijuana derivatives with higher ratios of therapeutic to undesirable effects.

THE NEED FOR MORE RESEARCH ON MARIJUANA

The explanation for all of these unanswered questions is insufficient research. We need to know much more about the metabolism of the various marijuana chemical compounds and their biologic effects. This will require many more studies in animals, with particular emphasis on subhuman primates. Basic pharmacologic information obtained in animal experiments will ultimately have to be tested in clinical studies on human beings.

Until 10 or 15 years ago, there was virtually no systematic, rigorously controlled research on the human health-related effects of marijuana and its major constituents. Even now, when standardized marijuana and pure synthetic cannabinoids are available for experimental studies, and good qualitative methods exist for the measurement of Δ-9-THC and its metabolites in body fluids, well-designed studies on human beings are relatively few. There are difficulties in studying the clinical effects of marijuana in human beings, particularly the effects of long-term use. And yet, without such studies the debate about the safety or hazard of marijuana will remain unresolved. Prospective cohort studies, as well as retrospective case-control studies, would be useful in identifying long-term behavioral and biological consequences of marijuana use.

The federal investment in research on the health-related effects of marijuana has been small, both in relation to the expenditure on other illicit drugs and in absolute terms. The committee considers the research particularly inadequate when viewed in light of the extent of marijuana use in this country, especially by young people. We believe there should be a greater investment in research on marijuana, and that investigator-initiated research grants should be the primary vehicle of support.

The committee considers all of the areas of research on marijuana that are supported by the National Institute on Drug Abuse to be important, but we did not judge the appropriateness of the allocation of resources among those areas, other than to conclude that there should be increased emphasis on studies in human beings and other primates. Recommendations for future research are presented at the end of Chapters 1-7 of this report.

CONCLUSIONS

The scientific evidence published to date indicates that marijuana has a broad range of psychological and biological effects, some of which, at least under certain conditions, are harmful to human health. Unfortunately, the available information does not tell us how serious this risk may be.

Our major conclusion is that what little we know for certain about the effects of marijuana on human health--and all that we have reason to suspect--justifies serious national concern. Of no less concern is the extent of our ignorance about many of the most basic and important questions about the drug. Our major recommendation is that there be a greatly intensified and more comprehensive program of research into the effects of marijuana on the health of the American people.

INTRODUCTION

The Institute of Medicine (IOM) of the National Academy of Sciences has undertaken this review and analysis of the health-related effects of marijuana* at the request of the Secretary of the Department of Health and Human Services (DHHS) and the Director of the National Institutes of Health (NIH).

Scientific controversy and public confusion about marijuana continue unabated and perhaps even are expanding, notwithstanding numerous reports on the topic from authoritative agencies and organizations (Fifth, Sixth, Seventh, and Eighth Annual Reports from the Secretary of Health, Education and Welfare to the Congress on Marijuana and Health; Fehr, et al., Cannabis: Adverse Effects on Health, 1980a; Tinklenberg, Marijuana and Health Hazards and Marijuana in the '80s, a report of the Council on Scientific Affairs, the American Medical Association, 1980). Increasing use of this substance and growing concern about its possible long- and short-term consequences for human health have added some urgency to the need for reassessment of the available data. Interest has been further heightened by recent suggestions that marijuana may also have some medical therapeutic value, which only intensifies the debate about what our public policy towards marijuana ought to be.

With this as background, the Secretary of Health, Education, and Welfare, Joseph A. Califano, Jr., in a press statement on April 18, 1979, announced the intention of his department to undertake a review that would ". . . assess the information and scientific work now available on the effects of marijuana." He followed that with a memorandum on May 16, 1979, to Donald S. Fredrickson, Director of NIH in which he further stated:

> This review must be undertaken by an independent scientific body that has not staked out a position in this highly controversial field. This review should be conducted by a

---

*The terms marijuana and cannabis will be used interchangeably in this report. Strictly speaking, they are not synonymous; cannabis is the more general term. (See Glossary, page 9.)

group of distinguished biomedical and clinical scientists and should involve thorough, systematic review and analysis of the research literature. . . . The report should identify the most urgently needed and promising lines of inquiry to build a firmer base for decision-making in years to come. The information should be available in a clear and incisive form for the general public.

While the Alcohol, Drug Abuse, and Mental Health Administration (ADAMHA) and its National Institute on Drug Abuse (NIDA) have provided leadership in research related to biological and health effects of marijuana, it is most important that we have a review by an independent nongovernmental body, such as the Institute of Medicine. In order to avoid even the appearance of a conflict of interest, inasmuch as this review will cover part of the research plan of ADAMHA-NIDA, I believe it is important that the National Institutes of Health serve as the responsible DHHS agency for seeing that such a review is conducted.

Following Mr. Califano's resignation, subsequent secretaries have confirmed to the Director of the NIH their desire to see this review carried forward. Accordingly, a contract between the NIH and the IOM was executed to provide for a study to commence September 30, 1980, and be completed by December 29, 1981.

THE COMMITTEE'S TASK

Under this contract, the IOM agreed to appoint a committee to:

1. analyze existing scientific evidence bearing on the possible hazards to the health and safety of users of marijuana;
2. analyze data concerning the possible therapeutic value and health benefits of marijuana;
3. assess federal research programs in this area;
4. identify promising new research directions, and make suggestions to improve the quality and usefulness of future research;
5. draw conclusions from this review that would accurately assess the limits of present knowledge and thereby provide a factual, scientific basis for the development of future government policy. Such an assessment also should be helpful to private citizens who want to make their own informed decisions about this subject.

The committee's charge specifically excluded the analysis or formulation of public policy.

PROCEDURE FOR THE STUDY

Primary responsibility for the conduct of the study was vested in a steering committee of 22 biologists, behavioral scientists, and clinicians. Although they all were experts in relevant disciplines, only a few had previously been involved in the study of marijuana or had taken public positions on the subject. The committee was divided into six panels, each concerned with major scientific areas: cardiovascular and respiratory system effects; neurobiological effects; epidemiological, behavioral, and psychosocial effects; reproductive biology and effects on the fetus; pharmacology, cell biology, and immunology; and genetic and oncogenic effects. Each panel was chaired by a member of the committee and usually had one or more additional committee members and several expert consultants, whose names appear in the front of this report. The committee also consulted with many other experts in the course of its work and received valuable help from many persons and organizations.

The full committee met five times to coordinate and assess its progress. In the intervals between these meetings, the panels held their own independent sessions and various ad hoc working groups met as necessary. The chairman and members of the committee staff were invited observers at the Conference on Adverse Health and Behavioral Consequences of Cannabis Use, which was sponsored by the Addiction Research Foundation (ARF) of Ontario and the World Health Organization (WHO) and held in Toronto, Canada, from March 30 to April 3, 1981. Other members of our committee served as working members of that conference. We were also fortunate in being able to work closely with members of the ARF/WHO conference staff and having access to all the documents prepared for the Canadian meeting as well as the revised draft of the summary report of the conference (1981).

The committee began by systematically reviewing all the literature published since 1975 on marijuana and related subjects, which had been collected by our staff through a Medline computer search. Earlier literature was selectively examined, as were a variety of other documents, reviews, and monographs on the subject. Our objective was not merely to compile and summarize, but also to evaluate the evidence critically and, with the aid of our consultants, form some judgment of the quality and reliability of the work. Our report is an assessment of what is and is not known, based on our best interpretations of the scientific literature. We confined our attention to published scientific articles as the primary sources of information, relying heavily on experts in each field to select the relevant papers and help us interpret the data.

To obtain additional information and opinions from the public and from professional groups on the health-related effects of marijuana, we solicited written responses in a notice in the Federal Register of February 24, 1981. Responses were received and incorporated into the records of the committee. (See Appendix A for a complete description.) The responses fell into three categories:

1. The dangers of marijuana. Letters in this category came from mothers whose children were using or had used marijuana. These parents believed that drug use by their children led to a lack of motivation and loss of interest in school and other activities. Letters about the harmfulness of the use of marijuana were also received from physicians and scientists.

2. <u>The therapeutic potential of marijuana.</u> Half of the responses were from people who used marijuana illegally for various medical problems and who urged that it be made easily available to patients. Several letters submitted by legislators and doctors described problems in obtaining marijuana for therapeutic use (see Appendix B). A group interested in the legitimate medical use of cannabis emphasized the need for continuing investigation into the numerous constituents of the marijuana plant for therapeutic uses.

3. <u>Support of general use and legalization of marijuana.</u> Letters were received from individuals and groups favoring the use of marijuana and actively promoting its legalization.

This report covers most of the concerns expressed by the public, except the question of legalization. The various statements included many opinions and much anecdotal evidence from laymen and scientists. The committee took note of this material, but has not cited any of it in this report unless it was supported by published data in the scientific literature.

THE ORGANIZATION OF THE REPORT

This report is divided into eight chapters and a summary. The summary includes the principal findings and conclusions of the study, together with suggestions for future research.

The first chapter reviews what is known about the chemistry and pharmacology of marijuana. Chapter 2 deals with the epidemiology and demography of the use of marijuana in the United States. The next three chapters discuss the effects of marijuana on cells, tissues, organs, and biological systems. Chapter 6 deals with behavioral and psychosocial effects. Chapter 7 discusses the present status of marijuana as a therapeutic agent. Chapter 8 describes and analyzes the federal research program on marijuana.

This report is intended to be intelligible to readers who are not expert on the subjects at hand. We have tried to use technical language only where accuracy would be compromised by less precise terms, and to keep the discussions as brief and as clearly stated as is consistent with our obligation to present a valid critique of the state of knowledge in this field. Although we have surveyed the literature as thoroughly as possible, our citations are selective rather than exhaustive, because they are intended to illustrate or document only the key points in the discussion. For comprehensive bibliographies, see Waller et al., 1976; Abel, 1979; and Kalant et al., 1980.

GLOSSARY OF TERMS FOR MARIJUANA-RELATED PRODUCTS

CANNABIDIOL (CBD) and CANNABINOL (CBN) are major cannabinoids generally present in cannabis (see CANNABIS and CANNABINOIDS).

CANNABINOIDS are a class of 21-carbon compounds present in Cannabis sativa. The basic structure contains a six-membered hydroaromatic ring and a benzene ring joined by a pyran moiety (see Figure 1-1 in Chapter 1). Derivatives include a number of carboxylic acids, their analogues, and transformation products.

CANNABIS is a general term for any of the various preparations of the plant Cannabis sativa and the cannabinoids obtained from it. "Cannabinoid" is a generic term for a class of compounds. Cannabis sativa, also called hemp, is an herbaceous annual plant that readily grows in temperate climates. Depending on the geographic region, and other considerations, the various natural preparations of cannabis possess different physical characteristics and concentrations of cannabinoids. Cannabis preparations may contain over 420 different compounds; of these, 61 have been identified as cannabinoids, many of which possess some biological activity. Marijuana, hashish, and tetrahydrocannabinol are examples of different forms or components of cannabis.

HASHISH is a resin, generally more potent than marijuana, which is obtained from Cannabis sativa by shaking, pressing, or scraping the leaves and flowers of the plant and usually contains some of the latter.

MARIJUANA is a general term for crude preparations obtained from the plant Cannabis sativa and is a mixture of crushed leaves, twigs, seeds, and sometimes the flowers of this plant. In the United States, the term "marijuana" has often been used interchangeably with cannabis to refer to any part of the plant or extract therefrom or any of the synthetic cannabinoids that induce somatic and psychic changes in man.

SINSEMILLA is a seedless variety of high-potency marijuana, originally grown in California.

TETRAHYDROCANNABINOL (THC) is one of the major groups of cannabinoids. Delta-9-THC is the principal active constituent in natural cannabis preparations. Delta-9-THC is also known as Δ-1-THC, by a different system of nomenclature. (In the United States, the Δ-9-THC content of marijuana ranges from unmeasurable amounts to about 6 percent.) Another active isomer, Δ-8-THC, is less often present in marijuana and typically occurs in minute amounts. Many derivatives of Δ-9-THC have been synthesized.

REFERENCES

Abel, E.L. A Comprehensive Guide to the Cannabis Literature Westport, Conn.: Greenwood Press, Inc., 1979.

American Medical Association. Marijuana in the '80s. Report of the Council on Scientific Affairs. Chicago Ill.: American Medical Association, 1980.

Fehr, K.O., Kalant, O.J., Kalant, H., and Single, E.W. Cannabis: Adverse Effects on Health. A statement prepared by the scientists of the Addiction Research Foundation of Ontario. Toronto: Addiction Research Foundation, 1980.

Kalant, O.J., Fehr, K.O., and Arras, D. <u>Cannabis: Health Hazards:</u>
<u>A Comprehensive Annotated Bibliography</u>. Toronto: Addiction
Research Foundation, 1980.

Report of Addiction Research Foundation/World Health Organization
(ARF/WHO). Conference on Adverse Health and Behavioral
Consequences of Cannabis Use. ARF/WHO, 1981.

Tinklenberg, J.R. (ed.) <u>Marijuana and Health Hazards: Methodological</u>
<u>Issues in Current Research</u>. New York: Academic Press, Inc.,
1975.

U.S. Department of Health, Education, and Welfare, Public Health
Service. <u>Marihuana and Health</u>. Fifth Annual Report to the
Congress from the Secretary of Health, Education, and Welfare,
1975. DHEW Publication No. (ADM)76-314. Washington, D.C.: U.S.
Government Printing Office, 1976.

U.S. Department of Health, Education, and Welfare, Public Health
Service. <u>Marihuana and Health</u>. Sixth Annual Report to the
Congress from the Secretary of Health, Education, and Welfare,
1976. DHEW Publication No. (ADM)77-443. Washington, D.C.: U.S.
Government Printing Office, 1977.

U.S. Department of Health, Education, and Welfare, Public Health
Service. <u>Marihuana and Health</u>. Seventh Annual Report to the
Congress from the Secretary of Health Education, and Welfare,
1977. DHEW Publication No. (ADM) 79-700. Washington, D.C.:
U.S. Government Printing Office, 1979.

U.S. Department of Health, Education, and Welfare, Public Health
Service. <u>Marijuana and Health</u>. Eighth Annual Report to the
Congress from the Secretary of Health, Education, and Welfare,
1980. DHEW Publication No. (ADM) 80-945. Washington, D.C.:
U.S. Government Printing Office, 1980.

Waller, C.W., Johnson, J.J., Buelke, J., and Turner, C.E.
<u>Marihuana: An Annotated Bibliography</u> New York: Macmillan
Information, 1976.

I

CHEMISTRY AND PHARMACOLOGY
OF MARIJUANA

The cannabis plant (<u>Cannabis sativa</u>) thrives under a variety of growing conditions. It has been cultivated for centuries, mainly for hemp fiber, but also for its psychoactive and putative medicinal properties (Abel, 1980; Turner et al., 1980). Although the behavioral and psychological effects were well described in literature of the nineteenth century (Kalant and Kalant, 1968), the complex chemistry and pharmacology of the cannabis plant discouraged extensive investigation until about 15 years ago.

The most prominent effects of cannabis are on psychological phenomena and behavior. Psychopharmacology and behavioral pharmacology have developed as divisions of scientific inquiry only over the past 25 years; therefore, the older cannabis literature, no matter how valuable for observations on other matters, does not provide a basis for quantitative pharmacological analysis and evaluation.

Early pharmacologists could work only with crude extracts of the plant. Although the general structure of the cannabinoids (Figure 1) was known by the turn of the century, the particular cannabinoids that were identified early and were available as pure substances were largely devoid of the characteristic psychoactive and other pharmacological effects of cannabis. Synthetic cannabinoids with cannabislike activity became available in the 1930s. It was not until 1964 that an active ingredient of cannabis was identified as Δ-9-tetrahydrocannabinol (THC) and synthesized (Figure 1) (Gaoni and Mechoulam, 1964; Mechoulam and Gaoni, 1965, 1967). In the mid-1960s, the isolation and synthesis of the main psychoactive component of cannabis and related cannabinoids, together with a rapid increase in the use of marijuana by middle class North American students, stimulated scientific activity (Waller et al., 1976; Waller et al., in press). This chapter, an overview of cannabis chemistry and pharmacology, emphasizes difficulties in the study of this drug (explored further in subsequent chapters) and in evaluating the literature.

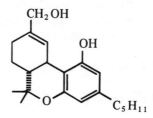

Δ-9-THC

Cannabinol

Cannabidiol

11-hydroxy-Δ-9-THC

FIGURE 1 Cannabinoid structures.

CANNABIS CHEMISTRY

Chemistry of the Plant

Cannabis, the crude material from the plant Cannabis sativa, contains
hundreds of chemicals. Most of these are found in other plants, but
61, termed cannabinoids, are unique to the cannabis plant (Table 1).
Natural and most synthetic cannabinoids are relatively insoluble in
water, but dissolve in fats and fat solvents and are therefore called
lipid soluble.

A single cannabinoid, Δ-9-THC, produces almost all the characteristic specific pharmacological effects of the complex, crude
cannabis mixtures. A number of synthetic cannabinoids have pharmacological effects similar to Δ-9-THC. Other cannabinoids in the
plant, for example, cannabinol (Figure 1), are almost inactive
pharmacologically or may interact with Δ-9-THC to modify its
actions. One cannabinoid, cannabidiol (CBD), can influence the
metabolism of another, Δ-9-THC (Siemens et al., 1976). A few
cannabinoids have effects quite different from Δ-9-THC. For
example, cannabidiol (Figure 1) has relatively little psychoactive
and cardiovascular effect but is an active anticonvulsant (Karler and
Turkanis, 1981).

Investigators have chemically altered the Δ-9-THC molecule in
an attempt to determine which of its structural elements are required
to produce behavioral or other effects (Mechoulam et al., 1980).
Studies of structure-activity relationships indicate that, to produce

14

TABLE 1 Chemical Constituents of Cannabis Preparations

1. Cannabinoids: <u>61 known</u>
   a. Cannabigerol (CBG) type: 6 known
   b. Cannabichromene (CBC) type: 4 known
   c. Cannabidiol (CBD) type: 7 known
   d. Δ-9-Tetrahydrocannabinol (Δ-9-THC) type: 9 known
   e. Δ-8-Tetrahydrocannabinol (Δ-8-THC) type: 2 known
   f. Cannabicyclol (CBL) type: 3 known
   g. Cannabielsoin (CBE) type: 3 known
   h. Cannabinol (CBN) type: 6 known
   i. Cannabinodiol (CBND) type: 2 known
   j. Cannabitriol (CBT) type: 6 known
   k. Miscellaneous types: 9 known
   l. Other cannabinoids: 4 known

2. Nitrogenous compounds: <u>20 known</u>

3. Amino acids: <u>18 known</u>

4. Proteins, glycoproteins, and enzymes: <u>9 known</u>

5. Sugars and related compounds: <u>34 known</u>

6. Hydrocarbons: <u>50 known</u>

7. Simple alcohols: <u>7 known</u>

8. Simple aldehydes: <u>12 known</u>

9. Simple ketones: <u>13 known</u>

10. Simple acids: <u>20 known</u>

11. Fatty acids: <u>12 known</u>

12. Simple esters and lactones: <u>13 known</u>

13. Steroids: <u>11 known</u>

14. Terpenes: <u>103 known</u>

15. Noncannabinoid phenols: <u>16 known</u>

16. Flavanoid glycosides: <u>19 known</u>

17. Vitamins: <u>1 known</u>

18. Pigments: <u>2 known</u>

SOURCE: Adapted from Turner, 1980.

effects on behavior, a pyran ring must be part of the three-ring system, a free phenolic hydroxyl on the aromatic ring at C-1, and a lipophilic side chain (C_5H_{11}) at C-3 (Figure 1). Understanding chemical structure-effect relationships is important to guide the synthesis of cannabinoids with differing pharmacological effects. Different effects of Δ-9-THC activity by chemical design will require further syntheses and pharmacological study of a large number of cannabinoids.

Chemistry of the Smoke

It is impossible to understand the effects of cannabis without quantitative control of the composition and the amount of the active substances, that is, control over the dose. Systematic pharmacology must therefore be performed using pure compounds. In the United States, cannabis usually is smoked, which complicates the pharmacology.

The smoke from any burning plant contains hundreds of chemicals that may have biological effects. This poses a dilemma for researchers, because consequences of smoking cannabis cannot be fully determined by studies only of the pure cannabinoids. Studies also are needed with doses of Δ-9-THC delivered, however imperfectly, by smoking.

The dose of Δ-9-THC obtained from smoking cannabis varies greatly, depending on many factors (Table 2). First, the content of Δ-9-THC depends on the genetic background or phenotype of the plant, the sex of the plant, conditions of growth and storage, and the plant preparation smoked. Second, much of the Δ-9-THC in fresh leaves that can be detected by gas-liquid chromatography (GLC) is in inactive carboxylated form. Decarboxylation to the active Δ-9-THC occurs slowly during storage and rapidly during heating, such as occurs in smoking or GLC analysis. Third, the way in which a cigarette is smoked can greatly affect how much of the Δ-9-THC content is absorbed by the smoker.

Cannabis smoke is similar to tobacco smoke in that it is a mixture of very small particles and a gas-vapor phase. Both the particulate and vapor phases contain many identified and probably some still unidentified constituents that, based on clinical experience with tobacco smoke, must be assumed to be potentially harmful (Leuchtenberger and Leuchtenberger, 1976). The amounts of some materials in tobacco cigarette and marijuana cigarette smoke are compared in Table 3. Toxic substances, such as carbon monoxide, hydrogen cyanide, and nitrosamines occur in similar concentrations in tobacco and marijuana smoke; so do the amounts of the particulate material known collectively as "tars."

It is not easy to compare the toxicity of a given number of marijuana cigarettes to a given number of tobacco cigarettes. There are general similarities in the composition of the smoke, but the variations in composition of both tobacco and marijuana cigarettes and differences in smoking techniques make simple extrapolations of risks of tobacco versus marijuana smoking not valid.

TABLE 2 Concentrations of Δ-9-THC in Different Varieties of Marijuana

Type	Percent Δ-9-THC (Percent by Weight)	Normalized Averages[e]
Nepal[c]	2.81	
Mexico[c]	1.68	1.00
Pakistan[c]	1.30	
Colombia[e]		3.00-3.50
India[f]	0.46 (grown above 2000 m)	
	1.39 (grown below 2000 m)	
Jamaica (Ganja)[h]	2.80 (mean)	
United States[c]	0.35	
Sinsemilla (fiber)[d]	0.21	
Sinsemilla (intermediate)[d]	3.58	
Sinsemilla (drug)[d]	6.28	3.00-11.00
Hashish (U.N. standard)[d]	2.22 (7.40)[b]	1.90
NIDA (cigarette 1)[d]	0.84	
NIDA (cigarette 2)[d]	1.86 (2.8)[g]	
Crude marijuana extract[g]	20.00	
Illicit hashish oil[g]	10.00-30.00 (up to 60)[a]	20.00
Research harvests[g]	0.90-2.80	

SOURCES: (a) Jones, 1980; (b) Braenden, 1972; (c) Turner, 1974; (d) Turner, 1980; (e) Turner, 1981; (f) Turner et al., 1979; (g) Rosenkrantz, 1981; (h) Marshman et al., 1976.

TABLE 3 Marijuana and Tobacco Reference Cigarette Analysis of Mainstream Smoke

	Marijuana Cigarette (85 mm)	Tobacco Cigarette (85 mm)
A. Cigarettes		
Average weight, mg	1115	1110
Moisture, percent	10.3	11.1
Pressure drop, cm	14.7	7.2
Static burning rate, mg/s	0.88	0.80
Puff number	10.7	11.1
B. Mainstream smoke		
I. Gas phase		
Carbon monoxide, vol. percent	3.99	4.58
mg	17.6	20.2
Carbon dioxide, vol. percent	8.27	9.38
mg	57.3	65.0
Ammonia, µg	228	199
HCN, µg	532	498
Cyanogen (CN)$_2$, µg	19	20
Isoprene, µg	83	310
Acetaldehyde, µg	1200	980
Acetone, µg	443	578
Acrolein, µg	92	85
Acetonitrile, µg	132	123
Benzene, µg	76	67
Toluene, µg	112	108
Vinyl chloride, ng[a]	5.4	12.4
Dimethylnitrosamine, ng[a]	75	84
Methylethylnitrosamine, ng[a]	27	30
pH, third puff	6.56	6.14
fifth puff	6.57	6.15
seventh puff	6.58	6.14
ninth puff	6.56	6.10
tenth puff	6.58	6.02
II. Particulate phase		
Total particulate matter, dry, mg	22.7	39.0
Phenol, µg	76.8	138.5
o-Cresol, µg	17.9	24
m- and p-Cresol, µg	54.4	65
Dimethylphenol, µg	6.8	14.4
Catechol, µg	188	328
Cannabidiol, µg	190	–
Δ^9-Tetrahydrocannabinol, µg	820	–
Cannabinol, µg	400	–
Nicotine, µg	–	2850
N-Nitrosonornicotine, ng[a]	–	390
Naphthalene, µg	3.0	1.2
1-Methylnaphthalene, µg	6.1	3.65
2-Methylnaphthalene	3.6	1.4
Benz(a)anthracene, ng[a]	75	43
Benzo(a)pyrene, ng[a]	31	21.1

[a]Indicates known carcinogens.
SOURCES: Hoffmann et al., 1975, 1976; Brunnemann et al., 1976, 1977.

Other Preparations

Besides the crude plant leaf material for smoking, usually called marijuana, resinous material from the plant, called hashish, and solvent extracts of the plant, termed hashish oil, sometimes appear on the illicit market. In many parts of the world, hashish is more commonly used than marijuana. As with all cannabis preparations, the Δ-9-THC content of hashish varies enormously, but the upper limits of Δ-9-THC content are usually much higher than for marijuana: 7 percent or higher and even higher for hashish oil (Table 2). However, even these generally more potent forms of cannabis may occasionally contain much less Δ-9-THC.

The mere designation of the nature of a cannabis preparation is an unreliable predictor of its Δ-9-THC content. The practical consequence of this for the clinical researcher is that the exposure to cannabis users is not known.

What Potency of Marijuana Is Available From Street Samples?

Because of the many confounding variables mentioned above, it is difficult to know what potency of psychoactive drug is in marijuana sold illicitly. The concentration of Δ-9-THC in a given sample will vary (Ritzlin et al., 1979). The content of Δ-9-THC from various street samples has been assayed. Marijuana from Drug Enforcement Administration confiscated samples; samples received through psychiatrists, police departments; and state crime laboratories, and fugitive* samples were quantitatively analyzed for Δ-9-THC and other cannabinoids. A physical description of the sample was made--e.g., buds, sinsemilla. The plants were also categorized by origin--where they were cultivated. The analysis showed that tremendous variability exists in the potency of Δ-9-THC on the street; normalized samples ranged from zero to 11 percent Δ-9-THC (Turner, 1981).

Analytic Methods

Detection and measurement of cannabinoids and their metabolites in body fluids is far more difficult than with such drugs as alcohol. The blood and tissue levels resulting from use of ordinary cannabis are very low--nanograms† per milliliter or lower. In addition, compounds like steroids, occurring normally in body fluids interfere with the measurement of cannabinoids in blood and can make the test much less sensitive than if pure cannabinoids in an uncontaminated

---

*Samples received, when no arrests were made.
†one billionth of a gram.

solution are being analyzed (Harvey et al., 1980; Harvey and Paton, 1980).

A combination of gas-liquid chromatography and mass spectrometry is the most sensitive direct method of measuring cannabinoids. That, however, requires skilled technicians and expensive equipment not readily available. Using modifications of this experimental technique, one can measure as little as 5 picograms* of Δ-9-THC in a milliliter of plasma (Harvey et al., 1980; Harvey and Paton, 1980). Radioimmunoassay and enzyme immunoassay techniques also are available, the lower limits of sensitivity of these methods now are not adequate for reliable measurements of Δ-9-THC in human blood more than a few hours after drug administration. A readily available enzyme immunoassay will detect cannabis metabolites in the urine for as long as a week after the smoking of a single marijuana cigarette. Thus, a positive urine test by this method is not necessarily indicative of use within the previous few hours and does not provide evidence of recent intoxication as a breath test does for alcohol. Assays for cannabinoids are likely to remain far more complicated than for alcohol and many other drugs.

PHARMACOLOGY OF CANNABIS

Implicit in a discussion of the effects of any drug is some determination of dose. The intensity and duration of effects in relation to drug dose must be determined or inferred from adequate pharmacologic study. The intensity and duration of a drug effect depends on at least three major factors:

1. The concentration of the drug at the sites of action in the body. This is determined by the dose, what the drug is dissolved in or mixed with, the route of administration, and the pharmacokinetics of the drug.
2. The sensitivity of the cells the drug acts upon.
3. The physiological state of the bodily systems being affected. This, in turn, depends on interactions with other systems and, especially for drugs with behavioral and psychological effects, as well as environmental and experiential factors, including the presence of other drugs.

With cannabis, many or even most of these factors are not always measurable or under the control of an investigator.

---

*1 pg = 10^{-12} grams.

Potency and Pharmacokinetic Considerations

Pharmacokinetic studies of the absorption, distribution, metabolism, and elimination of Δ-9-THC determine how long Δ-9-THC and its metabolites remain in the body. Pharmacokinetics vary with the route of drug administration and such factors as lipid solubility; Δ-9-THC tends to remain for long periods of time in fatty tissue.

When smoked, Δ-9-THC is rapidly absorbed by the blood in the lung. If taken orally, Δ-9-THC is not absorbed into the blood as rapidly. The rate of disappearance of Δ-9-THC from the blood varies with time (Lemberger et al., 1971a,b, 1972; Ohlsson et al., 1980). High blood levels fall rapidly for the first 30 minutes, as the Δ-9-THC distributes to tissues with high blood flow. After the initial distribution, the blood level falls much more slowly with a half-life* of 19 hours or more (Hunt and Jones, 1980). Metabolites[†] of Δ-9-THC have their own independent rates of elimination. Typically, metabolites are eliminated more slowly, having a half-life of approximately 50 hours (Hunt and Jones, 1980).

After an injection of a single dose of Δ-9-THC, approximately 25-30 percent of the compound and its metabolites remain in the body at 1 week (Lemberger et al., 1971b; Hunt and Jones, 1980). Essentially complete elimination of a single dose may take 30 days or longer (Jones, 1980). Thus, repeated administration of even small doses may lead to an accumulation of drug higher than levels reached at any time after a single dose.

Absorption

Inhaling smoke from a cannabis cigarette or pipe is pharmaco-kinetically different from ingesting cannabis. Smoking is a far more efficient way of delivering cannabinoids to the brain than ingestion because of the large surface area of the lungs. Inhaled, the cannabinoids in the smoke go rapidly from the lungs into the blood to the left side of the heart and are carried in seconds to the brain and other organs before passing through the liver. When smoked, a drug reaches the brain with relatively little time for metabolism or dilution. Many substances with high lipid solubility such as cannabinoids go quickly from blood into tissues, including brain tissues. Psychological and cardiovascular effects of cannabis are

---

*The half-life is a measure of how rapidly a drug is eliminated. It is the time required for the level of a drug to be reduced by one-half. If starting levels are ten units and the half-life is 24 hours, then 1 day after administration, the level will be 5 units, 2 days after administration 2.5 units, etc.

[†]There are more than 45 metabolites of major cannabinoids identified in different species, at least one of which, 11-OH-Δ-9-THC, is psychoactive.

evident within a few seconds of inhalation. Peak effects occur about
the time smoking is completed.

When taken by mouth, cannabinoids usually are in solutions or
suspensions. The material they are mixed with affects the rate of
absorption. For example, blood levels of Δ-9-THC were higher and
lasted longer when given in an oily solution than in an ethyl alcohol
solution (Perez-Reyes et al., 1973). This suggests that cannabis
eaten in food mixtures containing fat is better absorbed.

An important difference between smoking and ingestion is that
when cannabinoids are absorbed from the gut, the blood containing
them first goes directly through the liver. The liver rapidly clears
the Δ-9-THC from the blood and enzymatically changes much of the
Δ-9-THC to other metabolites before it reaches the brain (Hunt and
Jones, 1980). A large amount is metabolized to 11-hydroxy-Δ-9-THC
(Figure 1). It is unknown if the spectrum of effects of this
metabolite is identical to that of Δ-9-THC. When taken by mouth,
in contrast to when smoked, two or three times more Δ-9-THC is
required to obtain equivalent acute psychological and physiological
effects. After oral doses the effects develop more slowly, last
longer, are more variable, and cannot be controlled by the recipient
once the cannabis has been swallowed. In contrast, the smoker feels
the effects quickly and can modify inhalation at any time, although
overdosage is still possible. Unpleasant reactions to overdose are
more common following ingestion than inhalation.

A variety of other routes of administration have been used
experimentally in humans and in animals, including intravenous,
intraperitoneal, subcutaneous, intramuscular, topical (on the skin),
and into the conjunctival sac (eye). These various routes influence
the time to onset of effect, duration and peak intensity, and the
rate with which the effect disappears. Direct comparison of findings
in studies using differing administration routes is difficult and
must take these factors into consideration.

Human users of cannabis vary in their preferred routes of use.
In some countries and cultures cannabis is mainly taken by ingestion
(for example, India) and in others by inhalation (for example, the
United States). Because of the effects of route of administration on
pharmacology, it is reasonable to expect different health consequences
of the different routes of administration; therefore, comparisons of
health statistics among countries must be made with care.

Although smoking avoids many of the absorption problems discussed
above, a host of other variables affecting dose are introduced, such
as the size and packing of the cannabis cigarettes, the way the smoke
is inhaled, the number of puffs and the interval between puffs, the
temperature produced in the burning cigarette, and whether a cigarette
is shared. Because of the progressive concentration of cannabis
constituents in the cigarette butt, the last few puffs yield considerably more Δ-9-THC and particulate matter than do the earlier
puffs. All these and other factors affect the dose received, and
only rarely have they been measured. Only some of these factors are
under the conscious control of the cannabis smoker. About half of
the Δ-9-THC originally in a cannabis cigarette is lost by

combustion, by butt entrapment, in smoke not inhaled, and in smoke exhaled (Fehr and Kalant, 1972; Rosenkrantz, 1981).

It has been reported that, like nonsmokers of tobacco, individuals in a poorly ventilated room where cannabis is smoked may passively inhale active components (Zeidenberg et al., 1977). Because only trace amounts of cannabinoid metabolites are present in urine of these passive inhalers, it is unlikely that the low levels of the absorbed cannabinoids from the ambient air account for the so-called "contact high." Experiencing subjective cannabis effects in the presence of cannabis smokers could be explained by psychologic factors in addition to any pharmacologic ones. But, because studies have shown that children of parents who smoke tobacco are more likely to have respiratory infections during the first year of life--which may be due to their being exposed to cigarette smoke in the atmosphere (U.S. Department of Health, Education, and Welfare, 1979)--the issue of passive inhalation of marijuana smoke is worth further study.

Distribution

The lipid solubility of Δ-9-THC and other cannabinoids, including those with highest pharmacologic activity, facilitates distribution readily into tissues and cells throughout the body so blood levels drop rapidly. Initially, cannabinoid concentrations are highest in such tissues as lung, liver, and kidney that have a high blood flow (Agurell et al., 1969, 1970; Klausner and Dingell, 1971). Delta-9-THC crosses the placenta and enters the fetus of experimental animals (Kennedy and Waddell, 1972). Cannabinoid levels in the human fetus have not been studied. Small amounts are also found in the milk of experimental animals and can be transferred to progeny (Jakubovic et al., 1973; Chao et al., 1976). After initial distribution, concentrations of cannabinoids in tissues, cells, and subcellular compartments are highly nonuniform, determined no doubt by solubility and other physicochemical characteristics. Therefore, blood concentrations do not reflect concentrations at pharmacologically active sites, as they do with alcohol.

Metabolism and Elimination

Elimination of drugs and their metabolites is mostly through excretion by the kidney into the urine or by the gall bladder via the bile into the intestine and out with the feces. Cannabinoids do not pass out of the blood into the lungs and do not appear in breath in appreciable quantities. Some cannabinoids going into the intestine with bile are reabsorbed. Some also diffuse back through the kidney tubules during the process of urine formation, so the amounts finally excreted per unit of time are small. The net result of this recycling is that the cannabinoids are only slowly eliminated from the body.

Studies of the disappearance of Δ-9-THC from human plasma have
led to reports of values of half-lives that ranged from 19 hours in
experienced users (Hunt and Jones, 1980) to 57 hours in naive users
(Lemberger et al., 1971b). Whether this difference in half-life is
due to the experience of the user has not been established. Because
of their high lipid/water partition coefficients, Δ-9-THC and some
of its metabolites can be sequestered in fatty tissues. Following
the intravenous administration of radioactive Δ-9-THC to human
volunteers, however, 67 percent of the radioactivity was excreted in
1 week, 22 percent in the urine and 45 percent in feces (Lemberger et
al., 1971a). Almost no Δ-9-THC itself was excreted in the urine.
There may be fairly rapid and complete metabolism of free Δ-9-THC
followed by slow release and metabolism of sequestered Δ-9-THC and
retained metabolites. Because no direct measurements of cannabinoid
levels have been made in tissue samples from human cannabis users and
the data are limited in experimental animals, one can only infer from
blood levels what metabolites are accumulating and where.

In rats, after inhalation or intravenous administration of
radioactive Δ-9-THC, radioactivity persisted in the brain for at
least 7 days, mostly as metabolites (Ho et al., 1970). When given
subcutaneously in rats, even at intervals as great as a day or two
apart, Δ-9-THC will accumulate as metabolites (Kreuz and Axelrod,
1973). Accumulation of some cannabinoids with even less frequent
intake appears likely. Although most metabolites are concentrated in
fatty tissues, they will slowly pass into plasma and circulate though
all parts of the body, particularly including such organs as the
brain, and generally all membranes. The health consequences of the
continued presence of such foreign molecules are not known. The
marked persistence of the cannabinoids is quite unlike other widely
consumed agents, such as alcohol, nicotine, and caffeine, that are
rapidly metabolized and leave no trace a few hours after moderate
intake.

WHAT IS A LARGE OR SMALL CANNABIS DOSE?

Large and frequent doses of any drug are more likely to produce
adverse health effects than small infrequent doses of the drug.
Thus, judgments of health consequences of the use of cannabis can
only be made with implicit or explicit knowledge about dose. For the
reasons discussed above, the range of cannabinoid doses consumed
varies widely. Investigators usually report dose in terms of
marijuana cigarettes per unit of time, or they give some estimate of
the concentration of Δ-9-THC used for oral application. This is
not an adequate way to quantify the amount of cannabinoids actually
entering the body. Only one epidemiologic study provides a breakdown
of varying dose levels in excess of one cannabis cigarette daily
(Bachman et al., 1981). Epidemiologic surveys have not quantified
Δ-9-THC levels. When reporting less frequent use patterns than one
cigarette per day, investigators use measures that make it difficult
to compare studies. In this report, any general or average dose
estimates are approximations.

It is generally agreed that smoking five or six 1-gram cannabis cigarettes daily is a large dose (Dornbush et al., 1971; Rosenkrantz, 1981). Because of the variability of Δ-9-THC content of cannabis available from street samples, it would be more appropriate to consider this heavy use. The definition of a low dose is more controversial. Some consider one marijuana cigarette a day to be a large dose. Others think even one cigarette a week is regular, frequent, and a high dose.

With tobacco and alcohol, for which dose is easier to quantify, it took many years to establish what a small or large dose might be in terms of specifying doses that significantly increased the risk of various behavioral and health consequences. Even with those drugs, there is still disagreement as to precisely what a small and "safe" dose might be. There will be even more problems in specifying typical cannabis doses and predicting their likely health consequences.

In controlled laboratory conditions, ingested doses of more than 20 mg of Δ-9-THC generally are considered by both investigators and cannabis users to be large doses. Doses of less than 10 mg are considered small. Marijuana cigarettes containing more than 20 mg of Δ-9-THC seem to be a large dose, and those with 10 mg produce effects generally considered the result of a small dose. When volunteers were allowed to select their own self-determined smoked doses in controlled experiments, some smoked only one or two 20-mg cigarettes daily, while other similar volunteers smoked six to ten or more cigarettes per day. Variability in smoking patterns is great and not easily quantified; only broad range estimates of dose are possible.

GENERAL TOXICOLOGY

Delta-9-THC and related cannabinoids have very low lethal toxicity. That is, a very high single acute dose of Δ-9-THC is required to kill half of a population of experimental animals. This lethal dose for 50 percent of the animals is called the LD_{50}. The lack of well-authenticated cases of human deaths from acute Δ-9-THC or cannabis overdose is consistent with the experimental animal data. The lethal dose increases as the phylogenetic tree is ascended. The rat has an LD_{50} of 40 mg/kg intravenously, in contrast to a 125 mg/kg in the monkey (Rosenkrantz, 1981). Death is usually due to cardiac dysfunction. Delta-9-THC appears to be the most toxic of the cannabinoids.

Studies of chronic cannabis administration to animals have demonstrated delayed lethality. Animals die after several days of a repeated high dose (Rosenkrantz, 1981). The reason for this pattern is unclear. It could be related to accumulation of Δ-9-THC or metabolites in tissues.

A 1-year chronic treatment of rats with lower doses of cannabinoids produced a pattern of toxicity consisting of weight loss, pulmonary pathology when the drug is inhaled, and slowly developing behavioral toxicity characterized by hyperactivity, vertical jumping, fighting, and seizures (Rosenkrantz, 1981).

RELEVANCE OF NONHUMAN ANIMAL MODELS

Much of what is known about cannabis comes from experiments in animals. Some aspects of the pharmacology of any drug can only be studied in animals other than human beings. Findings from animal experiments have been criticized because of what were thought to be unreasonably high doses of cannabis given to the animals as compared with doses commonly used by human beings. Although extrapolation of human effects from animal data must be done with caution because of species differences in metabolic pathways and differing sensitivity and physiology, a blanket criticism of animal studies because of high doses is inappropriate. When an effect of a drug occurs consistently in several species, it is likely to occur in human beings. Comparisons of Δ-9-THC blood levels in human beings and in several species suggest roughly similar intensity of effects at similar blood levels in the various species (Rosenkrantz and Fleishman, 1979).

CANNABIS CONTAMINANTS

On occasion cannabis has been reported not only to contain the herbicide paraquat, but also salmonella bacteria and aspergillus fungus. Deliberate addition of such drugs as lysergic acid diethylamide (LSD), heroin, and phencyclidine (PCP) has been claimed. A plant material such as cannabis is not always handled in the most sanitary way, and a variety of contaminants are possible.

Paraquat

There is no question that large doses of paraquat by mouth or by aerosol can cause pulmonary fibrosis, but no cases in human beings have yet been proved to result from paraquat-contaminated cannabis. Few cannabis smokers are expected to be exposed to the large amounts of paraquat known to cause severe lung damage. This is not to say that no lung damage will occur from such exposure. A more extensive discussion of paraquat is in Appendix D.

Bacteria and Fungi

A few outbreaks of salmonellosis epidemiologically linked to marijuana use were reported from Ohio and Michigan (Schrader et al., 1981). Marijuana was found to be contaminated with the same type of salmonella that was obtained from the 62 patients experiencing diarrhea, fever, and abdominal pain.

Aspergillus, a fungus, is a common contaminant of some cannabis (Llewellyn and O'Rear, 1977; Llamas et al., 1978). The spores pass easily through contaminated marijuana cigarettes and when smoked are presumed to enter the body.

CELLULAR TOXICITY

A variety of effects on cellular processes have been reported, usually based on studies of _in vitro_ systems. The low water solubility of the cannabinoids and the need to add solvents and emulsifiers, along with a common tendency to use higher _in vitro_ concentrations than occurs in living animals, makes interpretation of such experiments difficult.

In related studies, Δ-9-THC alters the actions of a number of intracellular enzyme systems. The biological relevance of these drug/enzyme interactions is still unclear at this time, but, together with the cytotoxicity, it suggests that Δ-9-THC is producing marked effects on cell membranes and intracellular processes.

Almost nothing is known of the molecular mechanisms by which cannabinoids produce their effects in cells.

TOLERANCE AND DEPENDENCE

Repeated administration of most psychoactive drugs leads to the development of tolerance. This state of increased drug resistance results from two general mechanisms (Kalant et al., 1971):

- Dispositional tolerance resulting from lower drug concentrations at sites of action, usually because of increased rates of drug metabolism or elimination
- Functional tolerance arising from decreased sensitivity of the target cells.

Tolerance to most cannabinoid effects has been demonstrated both in animals and human beings (Jones, 1981). Tolerance can develop rapidly after only a few small doses. It disappears at an equally rapid rate for many effects, although after large doses in experimental animals some tolerance may persist for long periods (Jones, 1981). Systematic studies of tolerance loss have rarely been done. Many characteristics of tolerance to Δ-9-THC, particularly its pattern of rapid acquisition and loss, are similar to that occurring with opiates, nicotine, and cocaine (Jones, 1981). Most evidence suggests functional rather than dispositional means of acquiring tolerance.

The development of such tolerance to cannabis does not necessarily have health implications. However, if tolerance should lead to higher or more frequent doses, adverse consequences, e.g., respiratory effects, associated with higher usage could result.

Physical dependence, manifested by withdrawal signs and symptoms, can develop rapidly in animals and in human beings (Jones, 1981). The withdrawal syndrome is not life threatening. It is similar in many respects to the mild dependence produced by low doses of other sedatives. Withdrawal symptoms can include restlessness, irritability, mild agitation, insomnia, and sleep EEG disturbance.

Cannabis dependence does not mean the same thing as cannabis addiction. Dependence means only that a withdrawal syndrome can occur when drug taking is stopped. Addiction implies compulsive behavior to acquire the drug. The relationship between dependence and increased drug seeking or drug using is more theoretical than well documented, particularly in experiments with human beings. Given the appearance of tolerance and dependence with almost any psychoactive drug, it would be unusual not to find tolerance and dependence with the right dose and dosage schedule of cannabis. Good studies of the relationship of dependence, if any, to persistent drug use are important.

DRUG INTERACTIONS

Because cannabis often is consumed with other drugs, interactions can be expected. Other illicit drugs, tobacco, caffeine, alcohol, and over-the-counter or prescribed medications should be studied in combination with cannabis, because Δ-9-THC and its first metabolite are strongly bound to proteins in the plasma (Garrett and Hunt, 1974) and may interact with other drugs similarly bound. Cannabis and many other drugs share disposition by the hepatic metabolic enzyme systems, and there are possible interactions at the drug metabolism level. For example, drugs such as alcohol or pentobarbital can inhibit metabolism of Δ-9-THC by enzyme substrate competition. Or, if after a period of inhibition one drug is removed, the enzyme activity can increase so that faster than expected metabolism follows. If given simultaneously with other drugs, Δ-9-THC can slow metabolism of drugs such as theophyllin, antipyrine, ethanol, and pentobarbital (Benowitz and Jones, 1977; Jusko, 1979). Cannabidiol can also inhibit the metabolism of a variety of drugs normally metabolized by the shared hepatic enzyme systems.

Drug interactions also can occur by means of functional mechanisms. These can be additive, resulting in enhancement or prolongation of behavioral and psychological effects by cannabis when combined with other central nervous system depressant drugs, such as alcohol and barbiturates. Animals less tolerant to cannabis will also be less sensitive to other central nervous system depressants. This phenomenon is known as cross-tolerance. Drug interactions will be mentioned in subsequent chapters.

SUMMARY AND CONCLUSIONS

Cannabis is not a single drug, but a complex preparation containing many biologically active chemicals. The psychological and physiological effects produced by Δ-9-THC probably result from actions at sites within the central nervous system and elsewhere in the body, leading to the likelihood of complicated effects depending on dose, duration of use, and many other considerations.

The intensity of effect an individual experiences varies considerably according to the cannabis preparation and the amount taken, route of administration, frequency of use, and probably other not-well-recognized biological considerations. Dose variability must be considered both in conducting and in interpreting any studies of the effects of cannabis, particularly when trying to predict health consequences.

In research the use of pure Δ-9-THC avoids some problems of dose control but cannot provide a complete picture of cannabis effects, because the effects of Δ-9-THC in crude preparations of the plant may be influenced by other components. Other consequences of cannabis use, for example, exposure to harmful components in its smoke, will have deleterious health consequences in addition to anything produced by the Δ-9-THC.

The long persistence of cannabinoid metabolites in the body may have delayed effects or health implications not yet recognized, because, even with relatively infrequent use, there is chronic exposure to biologically unknown materials. In this respect, cannabis differs fundamentally from such drugs as alcohol, nicotine, and caffeine, which are rapidly metabolized and eliminated from the entire body.

Cannabinoid effects can be modified by many events, including interaction with other drugs and the development of tolerance. Both tolerance and dependence develop to many effects of the drug. The health significance of tolerance and dependence, particularly their importance in drug-seeking and drug-using behavior, has not been studied properly.

It is unlikely that adequate epidemiologic data will be available (soon) to enable good estimation of the health consequences of various usage levels.

A prerequisite is that adequate chemical analytical methods be applied on a large-scale basis to monitor actual exposures. Continued studies in experimental animals will play an essential role in the assessment of the health risks of cannabis. For example, the biological activities of Δ-9-THC metabolites can be assessed in experimental animals, but these tests are technically more difficult to do in human beings.

RECOMMENDATIONS FOR RESEARCH

Several research priorities are identified by the preceding discussion:

• Cannabinoids and their metabolites persist for relatively long periods in the body. More information is needed on the biological significance of that persistence in human beings. As a first step, the toxicological effects of the various metabolites need to be determined.

• Drug interactions alter the actions of cannabis. Cannabis use alters other drug effects. More information is necessary to make the combined effects of cannabis and other licit and illicit drugs more predictable, especially with respect to behavioral impairment and toxicity to lungs, liver, and other organs.

• Studies of the mechanism of action of cannabis should continue. Knowledge of mechanism is likely to provide powerful insights into the potential health effects.

• Improved chemical analytical methods are necessary. Epidemiologic appraisal of the health effects of cannabinoids requires methods suitable for wide-scale assays of exposures. Pharmacological verification of the self-reported extent of use will make experimental and clinical results much easier to interpret. A chemical "marker" of the frequent user would be useful. Screening techniques for the purpose of identifying and discouraging cannabis-impaired driving would also be valuable.

• Characterization of the toxicological significance of common cannabis contaminants such as paraquat and other chemicals, fungi, and bacteria should be continued.

• The development of tolerance is a factor that potentially modifies the expression of all psychoactive drug effects. Additional studies on the rates of acquisition and loss of tolerance and the relationship of these phenomena to dependence are necessary. The biological significance of the changes that underlie the development of tolerance should be established. The relationship, if any, between tolerance and dependence and drug-seeking behavior should be established.

• Cannabis products are variable and complex. More information on the amount, nature, and potency of the various preparations used around the world would facilitate calculations of exposures to its constituents. For example, what is the biological and toxicological significance of the minor components of cannabis smoke?

REFERENCES

Abel, E.L. Marihuana: The First Twelve Thousand Years. New York: Plenum Press, 1980.

Agurell, S., Nilsson, I.M., Ohlsson, A., and Sandberg, F. Elimination of tritium-labelled cannabinols in the rat with special reference to the development of tests for the identification of cannabis users. Biochem. Pharmacol. 18:1195-1201, 1969.

Agurell, S., Nilsson, I.M., Ohlsson, A., and Sandberg, F. On the metabolism of tritium-labelled delta-1-tetrahydrocannabinol in the rabbit. Biochem. Pharmacol. 19:1333-1339, 1970.

Bachman, J.G., Johnston, L.D., and O'Malley, P.M. Monitoring the Future. Questionnaire Responses from the Nation's High School Seniors, 1980. Ann Arbor, Mich.: Institute for Social Research, 1981.

Benowitz, N.L. and Jones, R.T. Effects of delta-9-tetrahydrocannabinol on drug distribution and metabolism. Clin. Pharmacol. Ther. 22:259-268, 1977.

Braenden, O.J. United Nations reference samples of cannabis, p. 193. In Paton, W.D.M. and Crown, J. (eds.) Cannabis and Its Derivatives. London: Oxford University Press, 1972.

Brunnemann, K.D., Lee, H.C., and Hoffmann, D. Chemical studies on tobacco smoke. XLVII. On the quantitative analysis of catechols and their reduction. Anal. Lett. 9:939-955, 1976.

Brunnemann, K.D., Yu, L., and Hoffmann, D. Chemical studies on tobacco smoke. XLIX. Gas chromatographic determination of hydrogen cyanide and cyanogen in tobacco smoke. J. Anal. Toxicol. 1:38-42, 1977.

Chao, F., Green, D.E., Forrest, I.S., Kaplan, J.N., and Winship-Ball, A. The passage of 14-C-Δ-tetrahydrocannabinol into the milk of lactating squirrel monkeys. Res. Commun. Chem. Path. Pharmacol. 15:303-317, 1976.

Dornbush, R.L., Fink, M., and Freedman, A.M. Marijuana, memory, and perception. Am. J. Psychiatry 128:194-197, 1971.

Fehr, K.O. and Kalant, H. Analysis of cannabis smoke obtained under different combustion conditions. Can. J. Physiol. Pharmacol. 50:761-767, 1972.

Gaoni, Y. and Mechoulam, R. Isolation, structure, and partial synthesis of an active constituent of hashish. J. Am. Chem. Soc. 86:1646-1647, 1964.

Garrett, E.R. and Hunt, C.A. Physicochemical properties, solubility and protein binding in delta-9-tetrahydrocannabinol. J. Pharm. Sci. 63:1056-1064, 1974.

Harvey, D.J. and Paton, W.D.M. Identification of in vivo liver metabolites of Δ-6-tetrahydrocannabinol produced by the mouse. Drug Metab. Disposition 8:178-186, 1980.

Harvey, D.J., Martin, B.R., and Paton, W.D.M. Identification of in vivo liver metabolites of delta-1-tetrahydrocannabinol, cannabidiol, and cannabinol produced by the guinea pig. J. Pharm. Pharmacol. 32:267-271, 1980.

Ho, B.T., Fritchie, G.E., Kralik, P.M., et al. Distribution of tritiated-1-delta-9-tetrahydrocannabinol in rat tissues after inhalation. J. Pharm. Pharmacol. 22:538-539, 1970.

Hoffmann, D., Brunnemann, K.D., Gori, G.B., and Wynder, E.L. On the carcinogenicity of marijuana smoke, pp. 63-81. In Runeckles, V.C. (ed.) Recent Advances in Phytochemistry. New York: Plenum Publishing Corp., 1975.

Hoffmann, D., Patrianakos, C., Brunneman, K.D., et al. Chromatographic determination of vinyl chloride in tobacco smoke. Anal. Chem. 48:47-50, 1976.

Hunt, A. and Jones, R.T. Tolerance and disposition of tetrahydrocannabinol in man. J. Pharmacol. Exp. Ther. 215:35-44, 1980.

Jakubovic, A., Hattori, T., and McGeer, P.L. Radioactivity in suckled rats after giving 14C-tetrahydrocannabinol to the mother. Eur. J. Pharmacol. 22:221-223, 1973.

Jones, R.T. Human effects: An overview, pp. 54-80. In Petersen, R.C. (ed.) Marijuana Research Findings: 1980. NIDA Research Monograph 31. DHHS Publication No. (ADM)80-1001. Washington, D.C.: U.S. Government Printing Office, 1980.

Jones, R.T. In Report of an Addiction Research Foundation/World Health Organization (ARF/WHO) Scientific Meeting on Adverse Health and Behavioral Consequences of Cannabis Use. ARF/WHO, Toronto, 1981.

Jusko, W.J. Influence of cigarette smoking on drug metabolism in man. Drug Metab. Rev. 9:221-236, 1979.

Kalant, O.J. and Kalant, H. Marihuana and its effects: An assessment of current knowledge. Addictions 15:1-7, 1968.

Kalant, H., LeBlanc, A.E., and Gibbons, R.J. Tolerance to, and dependence on, some non-opiate psychotropic drugs. Pharmacol. Rev. 23:135-191, 1971.

Karler, R. and Turkanis, S.A. Cannabinoids as potential antiepileptics. J. Clin. Pharmacol. 21:437S-448S, 1981.

Kennedy, J.S. and Waddell, W.J. Whole-body autoradiography of the pregnant mouse after administration of $^{14}C-\Delta-9-THC$. Toxicol. Appl. Pharmacol. 22:252-258, 1972.

Klausner, H.A. and Dingell, J.V. The metabolism and excretion of delta-9-tetrahydrocannabinol in the rat. Life Sci. 10:49-59, 1971.

Kreuz, D.S. and Axelrod, J. Delta-9-tetrahydrocannabinol: Localization in body fat. Science 179:391-393, 1973.

Lemberger, L., Axelrod, J., and Kopin, I.J. Metabolism and disposition of tetrahydrocannabinols in naive subjects and chronic marijuana users. Ann. N.Y. Acad. Sci. 191:142-154, 1971a.

Lemberger, L., Tamarkin, N.R., Axelrod, J., and Kopin, I.J. Delta-9-tetrahydrocannabinol: Metabolism and disposition in long-term marihuana smokers. Science 173:72-74, 1971b

Lemberger, L., Weiss, J.L., Watanabe, A.M., et al. Delta-9-tetrahydrocannabinol. Temporal correlation of the psychologic effects and blood levels after various routes of administration. N. Engl. J. Med. 286:685-688, 1972.

Leuchtenberger, C. and Leuchtenberger, R. Cytological and cytochemical studies of the effects of fresh marihuana cigarette smoke on growth and DNA metabolism of human lung cultures, pp. 595-612. In Braude, M.C. and Szara, S. (eds.) Pharmacology of Marihuana. New York: Raven Press, 1976.

Llamas, R., Hart, D.R., and Schneider, N.S. Allergic bronchopulmonary aspergillosis associated with smoking moldy marihuana. Chest 73:871-872, 1978.

Llewellyn, G.C. and O'Rear, C.E. Examination of fungal growth and aflatoxin production on marihuana. Mycopathologia 62:109-112, 1977.

Marshman, J.A., Popham, R.E., and Yawney, C.D. A note on the cannabinoid content of Jamaican ganja. Bull. Narcotics 26:63-68, 1976.

Mechoulam, R. and Gaoni, Y. A total synthesis of
Δ-1-tetrahydrocannabinol, the active constituent of hashish.
J. Am. Chem. Soc. 87:3273-3275, 1965.

Mechoulam, R. and Gaoni, Y. The absolute configuration of
Δ-1-tetrahydrocannabinol, the major active constituent of
hashish. Tetrahedron Lett. 12:1109-1111, 1967.

Mechoulam, R., Lander, N., Varkony, T.H., et al. Stereochemical
requirements for cannabinoid activity. J. Med. Chem.
23:1068-1072, 1980.

Ohlsson, A., Lindgren, J.E., Wahlen, A., et al. Plasma
delta-9-tetrahydrocannabinol concentrations and clinical effects
after oral and intravenous administration and smoking. Clin.
Pharmacol. Ther. 28:409-416, 1980.

Perez-Reyes, M., Lipton, M.A., Timmons, M.C., et al. Pharmacology of
orally administered delta-9-tetrahydrocannabinol. Clin.
Pharmacol. Ther. 14:48-55, 1973.

Ritzlin, R.S., Gupta, R.C., and Lundberg, G.D. Delta-9-
tetrahydrocannabinol levels in street samples of marijuana and
hashish: Correlation to user reactions. Clin. Toxicol.
15:45-53, 1979.

Rosenkrantz, H. The Immune response and marihuana, pp. 441-456. In
Nahas, G.G., Paton, W.D.M., and Idanpaan-Heikkila, J.E. (eds.)
Marihuana: Chemistry, Biochemistry, and Cellular Effects. New
York: Springer-Verlag, 1976.

Rosenkrantz, H. In Report of an Addiction Research Foundation/World
Health Organization (ARF/WHO) Scientific Meeting on Adverse
Health of Behavioral Consequences of Marijuana Use. ARF/WHO,
Toronto, 1981.

Rosenkrantz, H. and Fleischman, R.W. Effects of cannabis on lungs,
pp. 279-299. In Nahas, G.G. and Paton, W.D.M. (eds.) Marihuana:
Biological Effects. Analysis, Metabolism, Cellular Responses,
Reproduction and Brain Oxford: Pergamon Press, 1979.

Schrader, J., Steris, C., Halpin, T. et al. Salmonellosis traced to
marijuana--Ohio, Michigan. MMWR 30:77-79, 1981.

Siemens, A.J., Kalant, H., and deNie, J.C. Metabolic interactions
between Δ-9-tetrahydracannabinol and other cannabinoids in
rats, pp. 77-93. In Braude, M.C. and Szara, S. (eds.)
Pharmacology of Marihuana. New York: Raven Press, 1976.

Turner, C.E. Active substances in marijuana. Arch. Invest. Med.
Suppl. 5:135-140, 1974.

Turner, C.E., Cheng, P.C., Lewis, G.S., et al. Constituents of
Cannabis sativa. XV. Botanical and chemical profile of Indian
variants. Planta Med. 37:217-225, 1979.

Turner, C.E. Chemistry and metabolism, pp. 81-97. In Petersen, R.C.
(ed.) Marijuana Research Findings: 1980. NIDA Research
Monograph 31. DHHS Publication No. (ADM)80-1001. Washington,
D.C.: U.S. Government Printing Office, 1980.

Turner, C.E. Director, Research Institute of Pharmaceutical Science,
University of Mississippi, Oxford, Mississippi. Personal
communication, 1981.

Turner, C.E., Elsohly, M.A., and Boeren, E.G. Constituents of
Cannabis sativa L. XVII. A review of the natural constituents.
J. Natural Prod. 43:169-234, 1980.

U.S. Department of Health, Education and Welfare. Smoking and
Health: A Report of the Surgeon General. DHEW Publication No.
(PHS) 79-50066. Washington, D.C.: U.S. Government Printing
Office, 1979.

Waller, C.W., Johnson, J.J., Buelke, J., and Turner, C.E.
Marihuana: An Annotated Bibliography. New York: Macmillan
Information, 1976.

Waller, C.W., Nair, R.S., McAllister, A.F., et al. Marihuana: An
Annotated Bibliography. Volume 2 New York: Macmillan
Information (in press).

Zeidenberg, P., Bourdon, R., and Nahas, G.G. Marijuana intoxication
by passive inhalation: Documentation by detection of urinary
metabolites. Am. J. Psychiatry 134:76-78, 1977.

2

USE OF MARIJUANA
IN THE UNITED STATES

Epidemiologic studies provide information on the use of drugs in various subgroups of the population and on the changes in patterns of use over time. The epidemiologic approach is particularly useful in defining patterns of use of marijuana in American society and in describing and analyzing the behavioral and psychosocial antecedents and consequences of that use. One of the more difficult questions is whether particular behavior or effects that are associated with use of a drug are the consequences of that use, or whether attitudes, values, and behavior develop about the use of drugs to constitute factors that may actually lead to the use of drugs. One of the more useful epidemiologic study designs is a cohort study that follows the same individual with repeated observations at regular intervals over time. Such longitudinal studies have the potential for obtaining the most compelling evidence on the antecedents of known patterns of use of marijuana, as well as possible long-term psychosocial and biological outcomes for these individuals.

The committee, with the help of consultants, sought answers in the epidemiologic literature to the following five questions:

1. What are important patterns of use of marijuana in the American population including special groups?
2. What are the general characteristics of users of marijuana?
3. What is the profile of a user of marijuana on a "daily"* basis?
4. What is known about the antecedents of use of marijuana?
5. How is use of marijuana related to the use of other drugs?

The epidemiologic and survey literature have been extensively reviewed and the major longitudinal studies are summarized in a table in Appendix C. Much of our recent knowledge derives from two well-designed major, continuing nationwide monitoring efforts

---

*When placed in quotation marks, "daily" is used as defined by Johnston et al. (1980b), i.e., those individuals using marijuana 20 or more times in the preceding 30 days.

34

sponsored by the National Institute on Drug Abuse. One is based on general household population samples, the National Household Surveys. The second is based on populations of high school seniors and is called <u>Monitoring the Future</u>.

The National Household Surveys of the general population are conducted on an annual or biannual basis by Response Analysis Corporation and The George Washington University (Fishburne et al., 1980). There have been six cross-sectional studies since 1971. The latest one was in the winter of 1979-1980, and the next one will be initiated in 1982. The subjects are classified as youth (12-17), young adults (18-25), and older adults (26 and older). The questions relate to marijuana and other psychoactive drugs, including inhalants, hallucinogens, cocaine, heroin, stimulants, sedatives, and analgesics. Samples vary from about 3,000 to more than 7,200 new respondents at each survey. These are samples that document patterns of use of drugs in the specified populations at a given time.

<u>Monitoring the Future</u> (Johnston et al., 1980b) uses a cohort-sequential longitudinal design, in which a new cohort of high school seniors is surveyed each year, and a representative panel selected from that senior class is also followed over time in successive annual or biannual testings. The earliest panel has now been reinterviewed six times. This survey design makes it possible to disentangle antecedents from consequences of use as well as to distinguish changes due to increased age from changes due to cohort peculiarities or historical circumstances. Initiated in 1975 by the Survey Research Center of the University of Michigan, and directed by Lloyd Johnston and Jerald Bachman, the survey involves a question-naire self-administered each year by more than 16,000 high school seniors in 130 public and private schools throughout the United States, and longitudinal mail follow-ups of about 2,000 former students drawn, as panels, from each of the previously participating senior classes (Johnston et al., 1979a,b; 1980a,b).

Because the National Household Surveys and <u>Monitoring the Future</u> are surveys of persons in households or in high school, they exclude persons most likely to be using drugs--the transients, those without regular addresses, the school absentees or drop-outs, or those living in institutions or group quarters. These persons constitute a small proportion of the general population, and their exclusion does not significantly bias the epidemiologic estimates reported for the total population (Kandel, 1975a). However, data on the very heavy use of drugs may be underrepresented.

PATTERNS AND TRENDS OF USE OF MARIJUANA

General Population

The National Household Surveys found that marijuana was the most commonly used of all the nonlegal psychoactive drugs investigated, including inhalants, hallucinogens, cocaine, heroin, stimulants, sedatives, tranquilizers, and analgesics (Fishburne et al., 1980).

In 1979 more than 50 million persons had tried marijuana at least
once in their lives: 68.2 percent of young adults (18-25), or about
21 million; 30.9 percent of youth (12-17), or more than 7 million;
and 19.6 percent of older adults (26 and older), or 25 million. The
young adult age-group (18-25 years) has consistently showed the
highest rates of current use (used in past month) and ever use
(lifetime prevalence), and the older adult groups (26 and older) had
the lowest user rates. Male users outnumbered females in all age
groups. Between 1977 and 1979, significant increases in current use
and ever use of marijuana were observed among the young adult and
older adult cohorts (Figure 2). In 1979, in the young adult cohort,
the most significant increases in use in the past month were found in
males, whites, high school nongraduates, people in the southern
United States, and those living in nonmetropolitan areas. In the
older adult groups, the most significant recent increase in current
use of marijuana was observed in males, whites, college graduates,
and people living in the southern states (Miller and Cisin, 1980).

In the early 1960s, illicit drug use in the United States was
chiefly a phenomenon of large coastal cities. But since then, rates
in other regions of the country and in cities of all sizes have
rapidly increased until patterns of use are becoming increasingly
comparable for all sectors in the United States. At current levels
of use, some experience with marijuana in adolescence is becoming the
norm rather than the exception throughout the United States. Other
major survey studies have confirmed the findings of the National
Household Survey for comparable cohort populations (Gallup Opinion
Index, 1976; O'Donnell et al., 1976).

Military Personnel

Much attention has recently been focused on what appear to be high
rates of use of illicit drugs among military personnel. Studies of
drug use among male army veterans of the Vietnam War in 1972 showed
that marijuana was the most commonly used illicit drug before and
after the war (Robins, 1974). A random sample of 470 men was selected
from the 13,760 enlisted men who returned to the U.S. in September
1971. Of the 451 men who were interviewed, 69 percent had used
marijuana while in Vietnam, with 28 percent stating this was their
first use of the drug. The lifetime prevalence of use of marijuana
was 41 percent prior to Vietnam; 45 percent of the veterans reported
using marijuana in the 10 months following return to the United
States. Among this group the prevalence of weekly use doubled from
12 percent prior to Vietnam to 25 percent following the war.

A worldwide survey of nonmedical use of drugs and alcohol among
U.S. active duty military personnel was conducted in 1980 under the
sponsorship of the U.S. Department of Defense (Burt et al., 1980).
In an anonymous, self-administered questionnaire given to a representative sample of more than 16,000 persons, marijuana was found to
be the most commonly used illicit drug. Twenty-six percent admitted
to having used "marijuana/hashish" within the past 30 days and 35

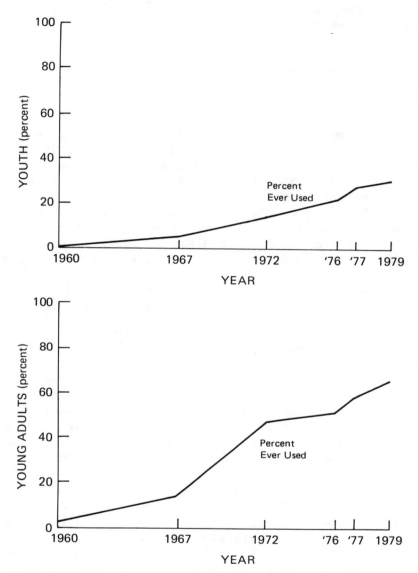

FIGURE 2 Marijuana: trends in lifetime experience, youth, and young adults. Adapted from J.D. Miller and I.H. Cisin. <u>Highlights from the National Survey on Drug Abuse: 1979</u>. Washington, D.C.: U.S. Government Printing Office, 1980. Youth = 12 to 17 years old; young adults = 18 to 25 years old.

percent to having used it in the past 12 months. Five percent of the sample reported use of marijuana daily.

When users of drugs were itemized according to military pay classifications, the largest percentage of current use of marijuana was in the lowest ranks of the military.

Adolescents and Young Adults

Patterns and Trends

One of the compelling reasons to focus on adolescence in studying marijuana is the pervasive and increasing use by this age group. As was mentioned earlier, in 1980 all geographical regions of the United States and all socioeconomic classes had high and increasingly comparable involvement in use of marijuana.

The year 1960 has been taken as a baseline year that represents the stable level of overall use of marijuana that had characterized the United States for most of its history. Figure 2 shows the trends for use of marijuana from 1960 through 1979, revealing the sharp upward climb of use of marijuana starting in 1967. The dramatic rise in use of marijuana by adolescents has recently slowed, and the lifetime prevalence rates (ever use) of marijuana have remained at approximately 60 percent of all high school seniors for the years 1979 and 1980 (Figure 3). To put it another way, in 1979 over 2.5 million high school seniors had tried or were users of marijuana. (This figure is derived from calculations based on 1979 Census Bureau data that give a figure of 4,276,000 for number of 18-year-olds in the population. The committee is aware that all 18-year-olds are not high school seniors and that such a calculation may underreport the numbers of users of marijuana, particularly heavy users who have been shown to be more likely to have dropped out of school. Similar calculations have been attempted throughout this chapter.)

The use of other types of drugs by young people also increased beginning in 1967 (Miller and Cisin, 1980). Figure 4 gives the most recent nationwide figures for use of 11 types of drugs among American high school seniors (average age 18 years). With the exception of negligible use of heroin, the figures for use of all other drugs are substantial. Increases in patterns of use have not been as dramatic for other drugs (except for recent cocaine increases) as they have been for marijuana. Use of marijuana, tobacco, and alcohol far outstrips that of all other drugs. In 1980 the lifetime prevalence (ever use) for these substances by high school seniors was marijuana--60 percent, tobacco--71 percent, and alcohol--93 percent.

Of even greater interest are the percentages of high school seniors who use the 11 types of drugs "daily." In 1980 marijuana was used "daily" by 9.1 percent (about 390,000), alcohol by 6.0 percent (about 256,000), and tobacco cigarettes by 21.3 percent (about 900,000) of high school seniors (Johnston et al., 1980a). No other substance was used that frequently by as many as 1 percent of the

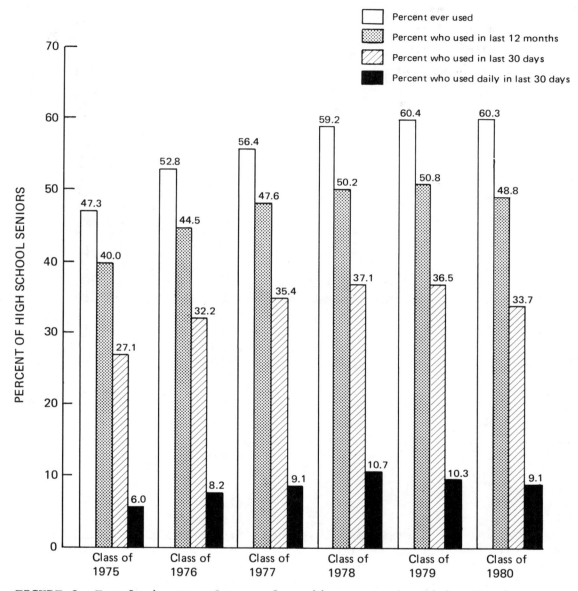

FIGURE 3 Trends in prevalence of marijuana use by high school
seniors, 1975-1980 (in school). Adapted from L.D. Johnson, J.G.
Bachman, and P.M. O'Malley, Highlights from Student Drug Use in
America, 1975-1980. DHHS Publication No. (ADM) 81-1066. Washington,
D.C.: U.S. Government Printing Office, 1980a.

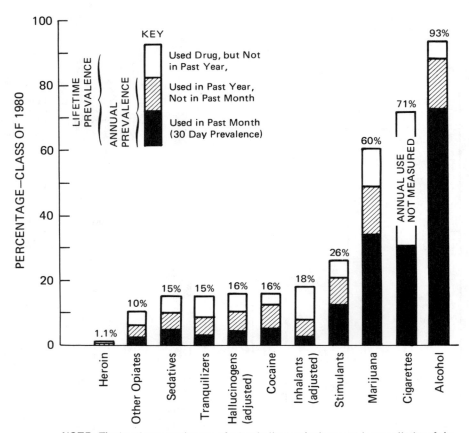

NOTE: The bracket near the top of a bar indicates the lower and upper limits of the 95% confidence interval.

FIGURE 4 Prevalence and recency of use. Eleven types of drugs, class of 1980. SOURCE: Johnson, L.D., Bachman, J.G., and O'Malley, P.M. Highlights from Student Drug Use in America, 1975-1980. DHHS Publication No. (ADM) 81-1066. Washington, D.C.: U.S. Government Printing Office, 1980a.

students. These figures show that legal (for adults) drugs are used much more frequently than illegal ones. Reports of illegal use of drugs show that experimentation with marijuana has, by far, the highest prevalence. It should be noted, also, that "daily" use of marijuana (9 percent) among high school seniors is now more prevalent than "daily" drinking (6 percent) of alcoholic beverages.

In 1980, for the first time since 1975, when the Monitoring the Future data collection began among high school seniors, the percentage of "daily" users of marijuana among seniors in high school declined significantly from 10.3 percent in 1979 to 9.1 percent in 1980 (Figure 3), and there was a leveling of lifetime prevalence at approximately 60 percent. Furthermore, the proportion of current users among those who ever used marijuana also showed a statistically significant decline in 1980 as compared to 1979, from 60 percent to 56 percent. However, "daily" users may be increasingly underrepresented in recent senior high school classes due to absenteeism and drop-out associated with increasingly earlier and extensive involvement in use of marijuana. The extent to which long-term "daily" users have dropped out of school by the senior year of high school cannot be ascertained from monitoring the future. Kandel (1975a) found that absentees differed from students attending school regularly. Fifty-six percent of absentees reported use of marijuana as compared to 38 percent of in-class students. Studies that document the patterns of marijuana use in school drop-outs are needed.

Correlates of Use

Overall levels of use of marijuana have been shown to correlate with patterns of use of the drug.

   1.   Increased prevalance is associated with younger age of initiation into use of marijuana. As successive cohorts of high school seniors have shown increasingly higher levels of experience with marijuana from 1975 through 1980, these cohorts also report increasingly earlier ages at first use of marijuana. For example, in the senior class of 1980, which had a lifetime prevalence of 60 percent by senior year, 25 percent of those using marijuana had begun in the eighth grade (average age 14) or below. In 1975 when lifetime prevalence was 47 percent, 15.3 percent of marijuana users had begun in eighth grade or below. It is of some interest to compare reported age of use of marijuana by grade for the senior class of 1980 (lifetime prevalence 60 percent) and alcohol (lifetime prevalence 93.2 percent). The more prevalent drug, alcohol, is used at earlier ages than marijuana. Thirty-three percent of alcohol users had started at eighth grade as compared to 21.5 percent of marijuana users (Johnston et al., 1980a).
   2.   Earlier onset of use of any drug is associated with greater involvement in use of all other drugs. The earlier the introduction to legal (for adults) drugs, the greater the probability that the adolescent will also experiment with illicit drugs. For example, among young adults 18-25 years of age surveyed from the general population in 1979-1980, the proportion who had experimented with any illicit drug other than marijuana ranged from 87 percent among those who reported having first tried alcohol or marijuana at ages 13 or 14, to 47 percent among those who first tried these drugs at ages 15-17, and 5 percent among those who first experimented at age 18 or over (Rittenhouse, 1980). The finding that the earlier the experimentation with marijuana, the greater the intensity of involvement and the greater the likelihood of using more serious drugs has been confirmed in many studies (e.g., Miller and Cisin, 1980; Johnston et al., 1980a; Kandel et al., 1981).
   3.   Greater overall prevalence of use of marijuana is associated with greater persistence of use of marijuana into later years of adult life. The current prevalence rates for use of marijuana by persons in their mid-30s are increasing (Cisin et al., 1978). Many

studies have not sampled this population in the belief that use of marijuana drops off sharply in the mid-20s. Among males, the prevalence rate for use of marijuana in the past month for over-26-year olds went from 4 percent in 1977 to 9 percent in 1979. It will be exceedingly important to monitor the trends in all older adult age groups.

Marijuana and the Use of Other Drugs

One of the key questions asked over the years is, does marijuana lead to the use of other drugs. In any population, the use of various drugs appears interrelated and users of any type of drug, whether legal or illegal, are much more likely to use other types of drugs than nonusers. For example, young people who smoke tobacco are also much more likely to have used alcohol or marijuana than nonsmokers (Fishburne et al., 1980). Similarly, there is a strong association between the use of marijuana and of other illicit drugs. Young people who use marijuana are more likely to be consuming other substances, such as alcohol and tobacco, as well as other illicit drugs (Johnston et al., 1980b). The association increases with extent of marijuana involvement and is especially striking among those young people who use marijuana on a "daily" basis, as will be discussed below.

Results from the National Household Surveys and from samples of high school seniors had indicated that the ratio of rates of use of illicit drugs other than marijuana to use of marijuana declined through 1979 (Kandel, 1980; Miller and Cisin, 1980). In 1980, however, the ratio started to rise again. Thus, in 1980, 65 percent of marijuana users among the high school seniors had also used other illicit drugs as compared to 61 percent in 1979 (Johnston et al., 1980a).

"Daily" Users in High School

Because any health risks resulting from the use of marijuana would be most likely to appear first in chronic users of the drug, the young persons who are chronic and heavy users are of special interest. The committee reports in some detail the findings on this group. The ranks of "daily" users are large. In 1980 they represented more than 9 percent of high school seniors or over 390,000 18-year-olds in the United States. One out of 11 seniors fitted the definition of "daily" users (20 or more occasions of reported use within the preceding 30 days). Collection of systematic data on such users began in 1975 with the annual monitoring of in-school high school seniors. There are many gaps in our knowledge about this group, but sufficient data have been accumulated that it is now possible to describe many of the behavioral attributes of the "daily" users. Most of these data come from Monitoring the Future. Some of the findings recently reported by Johnston (1980, 1981) and Bachman et al. (1981) are as follows:

Demographic Findings

Rates of "daily" use do not vary among regions of the country, but "daily" use shows a strong positive relationship to the size of the community and is more prevalent in urban areas. Males are "daily" users at almost double the rate of females (13 percent versus 7 percent). "Daily" use among white students is double that for blacks (11 percent versus 5 percent). "Daily" use is spread evenly across socioeconomic levels as defined in terms of parents' education. "Daily" use is only slightly higher among those from homes in which one or both parents are absent.

Academic Performance and Goals

"Daily" use is associated with poor school achievement. Among non-college-bound seniors the rate of "daily" use is almost double that found among the college-bound (13 percent versus 7 percent). There are strong and positive correlations of "daily" use and cutting classes, school absences, and truancy.

Much of "daily" use takes place within the school setting. A statewide study of seventh through twelfth grade pupils in New York, conducted in 1978 by the New York State Drug Abuse Commission, found that 50 percent of those using marijuana within the last 6 months had been intoxicated one or more times while in class (Johnson and Uppal, 1980). In contrast, alcohol tends to be used most frequently after school and on weekends.

Religious Commitment

A commitment to religion and self-ratings of strong belief in law-abiding behavior are associated with lower than average rates of "daily" use.

Dating and Social Life

Dating and social life show strong relationships with "daily" use of marijuana. Those who spend more time on dates have the highest rates of "daily" use of marijuana. Among those students who go out 6 or 7 nights a week and are practically never at home, 34 percent are "daily" marijuana users.

Use of Other Drugs

"Daily" marijuana users are much more likely than their peers to be extensive users of other drugs. Thus, of seniors in the class of 1979, 27 percent of "daily" users of marijuana drank alcohol as frequently, versus 7 percent for the age-group as a whole; and 59 percent of "daily" users of marijuana smoked cigarettes as frequently versus 25 percent for the group as a whole (Johnston et al., 1980b).

With respect to use of other illicit drugs, the rates for "daily" users of marijuana generally run five to seven times the average for the age group as a whole; 47 percent of "daily" users are current* users of amphetamines; 31 percent of cocaine; and their current usage figures run from 15 to 17 percent for barbiturates, for lysergic acid diethylamide (LSD), for phencyclidine (PCP), for methaqualone, and for tranquilizers. Since nearly two-thirds of daily marijuana users (64 percent) are current users of hashish, they have substantial exposure to a high-potency form of marijuana.

We also know from data on age at first use that many of these "daily" marijuana users began their use of cigarettes, alcohol, and various other illicit drugs at quite an early age. To illustrate, by the end of eighth grade 40 percent of them had smoked cigarettes "daily" and 50 percent had taken their first drink. Just about half of them (48 percent) first tried marijuana by the eighth grade, and most of the remainder (another 30 percent) started in ninth grade. These are very early ages of initiation for all three drugs. Similarly, these youngsters tend to take up the other illicit drugs at an earlier than average age—though most of that use still is initiated after ninth grade. "Daily" use tends to persist longer into adult life than anticipated. In 1979, 4 years after graduation from high school, 51 percent of marijuana users of the senior class of 1975 were still "daily" users and an additional 34 percent were current although not "daily" users (Johnston, 1980).

"Daily" Users After High School

Using a national sample of 19- to 22-year-olds derived from the follow-up surveys of <u>Monitoring the Future</u>, Johnston (1981) reported on "daily" use of marijuana after high school. (These findings are reproduced nearly verbatim below.)

College Student Status

Student status after high school correlates negatively with "daily" use; that is, full-time college students have the lowest rate (8 percent), part-time students the next lowest (10 percent), and nonstudents the highest rate (13 percent). However, although full-time students have a lower than average rate of "daily" use, they showed the greatest increase after high school (up from 4.5 to 8.3 percent): they simply started from a very low level and in a sense were "catching up."

---

*A current user is one who has used the drug in the thirty days preceding the surveys.

Living Status

Young people who are living away from home have a higher proportion of "daily" use than those still living with their parents (12 percent versus 10 percent), probably reflecting the result of reduced social control by parents. Those who remained living with their parents (nearly half) showed relatively little increase in use (up 1.3 percent), while those who moved out increased their daily use rate substantially (up 3.9 percent).

Marital Status

Those who are single are almost twice as likely to be "daily" users as those who are married (11.4 percent versus 6.6 percent), and those without children are somewhat more likely to use marijuana than those with children (11 percent versus 8 percent). It appears that these role responsibilities have a dampening effect on use. In the face of an overall 2.6 percent increase in "daily" prevalence after high school for the whole sample, those who were married showed virtually no increase (up 0.2 percent) and those with children actually had a decline in use (down 1.5 percent).

Type of dwelling

"Daily" use is highest for those living in a rented room (14 percent) or apartment (12 percent), and lowest for those living in a college dorm (8 percent). Obviously one's dwelling arrangement is highly correlated with his or her major activity after high school, as these differences reflect.

Employment

Employment status is unrelated to "daily" use. For those in military service, "daily" use dropped slightly after high school (from 13.4 percent to 12.4 percent). The activity group with by far the lowest "daily" use rate are the full-time homemakers (4 percent), which certainly occurs, in part, because they nearly all are female, married, and in many cases have young children.

Reasons for Using or Abstaining

Reasons for "Daily" Use of Marijuana

What reasons do "daily" users give for their use of marijuana? They tend to use marijuana to produce an intoxicated feeling, to cope psychologically with feelings of distress, to augment the effects of other drugs, and to participate in drug-using friendships. On a checklist of 13 possible reasons, nearly all of the seniors who were "daily" users checked "to feel good or get high" (94 percent) and "to have a good time with my friends" (79 percent). Two-thirds said they used it to relax (67 percent) and nearly half said they used it to relieve boredom (45 percent). Roughly a quarter of the "daily" users checked each of the following: "to get away from my problems" (27 percent), "because of anger or frustration" (23 percent), and "to get through the day" (22 percent). These psychological coping motives in particular seem to distinguish the "daily" users from the less frequent users. A fairly high proportion (30 percent) also said that they used marijuana to increase the effects of other drugs, while only 10 percent of the other current users gave this reason. Only 11 percent of the "daily" users, or 1 percent of the total sample, stated that they used it because they felt "hooked" or had to have it. All of these responses for seniors were closely replicated among the "daily" users in the 19- to 22-year-old sample (Johnston, 1981).

Nearly all "daily" users (over 85 percent), whether in high school or past high school, say (1) that most or all of their friends smoke marijuana, (2) that most or all of their friends drink alcohol, (3) that more than a few of their friends get drunk every week, (4) that more than a few of their friends smoke cigarettes, and (5) that at least a few of their friends use a number of other illicit drugs. This degree of immersion in a drug-using friendship circle contrasts sharply to what we observe for their peers, even those who are current but less frequent users of marijuana. Clearly the social supports and the social pressures are there, both during and after high school, for the "daily" user to continue his or her habit.

Reasons for Quitting and Abstaining

A number of users of marijuana stop using the drug (Johnston, 1981). Among students (in the classes of 1978 through 1980 combined), those who have used marijuana 40 or more times but have stopped by their senior year give as their most commonly mentioned reason on a comprehensive list of 17 reasons that "they don't feel like getting high" (56 percent mentioned). Also frequently mentioned, however, are concerns about possible physical effects (41 percent); concern about possible psychological effects (38 percent); and, more specifically, concern about loss of energy or ambition (41 percent). These reasons also ranked high among those young people who smoked less than 40 times before they stopped, as did two additional reasons--concern about parental disapproval and finding that use of marijuana was not intrinsically enjoyable.

Concern about possible health effects appears to play a role in young people's giving up the drug and is mentioned considerably more often among quitters now than in 1976. Concern about physical health increased substantially between 1976 and 1980 among all high school seniors, from 35 percent to 57 percent, while concern about psychological damage went from 34 percent to 53 percent. A similar analysis of the reasons given for abstaining by the minority (about

40 percent) of seniors who have never tried marijuana reveals concern about physical (71 percent) and psychological (68 percent) consequences, which are mentioned far more often than any other type of reason. Social or ideological constraints or disinterest in getting high are infrequently mentioned. There also has been a significant increase in health concerns among the abstaining segment since 1976, though not as large as among quitters.

In summary, many "daily" users themselves see some negative consequences of their habit, and there perhaps are some consequences of which they are unaware. The fact that the "daily" smoking of marijuana is proving to be more enduring and stable than many may have thought increases the probability of cumulative, long-term effects. The fact that so many young people are becoming "daily" users now puts a substantial number of people at risk of whatever the long-term consequences may prove to be.

Sequence of Drug Use

Regardless of the age of onset, there is a predictable sequence in the patterns of initiation into the use of available drugs. Independent longitudinal studies have confirmed and identified a stable sequence of drug use (Hamburg et al., 1975; Kandel, 1975b; Kandel and Faust, 1975). The legal drugs for adults, such as alcohol and tobacco, are an early, integral, and crucial part of the sequence. Their use precedes the use of all illicit drugs. At least four distinct successive stages of adolescent involvement with drugs can be identified: (1) use of beer or wine, (2) use of tobacco cigarettes or hard liquor, (3) use of marijuana, and (4) use of other illicit drugs (Kandel, 1975b). A fifth stage, problem drinking, may take place between marijuana and other illicit drugs (Jessor et al., 1980). Adolescents rarely proceed from beer and wine to illicit drugs without use of either hard liquor or tobacco cigarettes as an intermediate step. Furthermore, there is an additive effect such that the highest proportion of adolescents who move to marijuana are those who have experience with both hard liquor and tobacco. For example, among 12- to 17-year-olds in the general population, the proportion who have ever experimented with marijuana is 81 percent among current tobacco cigarette smokers as compared to 24 percent among nonsmokers (Fishburne et al., 1980). However, position on a particular point in the sequence does not indicate that the young person will necessarily progress to other drugs higher up in the sequence. Participation in each stage is a necessary but not sufficient condition for participation in a later stage. There is no evidence to support the belief that the use of one drug will inevitably lead to use of any other drug. In other words, persons at the top of the ladder of use of drugs typically will have used all substances at lower levels, including marijuana. However, those at lower rungs may stay there and not move to higher rungs of the ladder.

For example, data from the National Household Surveys (Fishburne et al., 1980) indicate that of those 18-25 years old who have tried marijuana, almost all are users of tobacco or alcohol; however, only slightly more than one-fourth of this 18- to 25-year-old population report having gone on to try any illegal drug other than marijuana. Of those who try other illegal drugs, only a very small percentage report being current users (Fishburne et al., 1980).

Although it is of great interest, relatively little is known about the factors that determine which persons will choose to go through the sequence of drug use or the rapidity with which they will do so. Existing research gives us some clues that users of illicit drugs possess some distinguishing features.

There are four clusters of variables--parental influences, peer influences, adolescent involvement in deviant behaviors, and adolescent beliefs and values--that assume differential importance for predicting involvement at each stage of drug behavior (Kandel et al., 1978a,b).

Involvement with drugs legal for adults is the earliest level of drug use. Adolescents who start to drink are exposed to peers and parents who drink, suggesting that these youths learn drinking patterns from their parents. Adolescents who have engaged in a number of delinquent or deviant activities, and who seek high levels of sociability with their peers are likely to become involved with alcohol. Similar patterns are found with tobacco smoking, also one of the earliest drugs to be tried.

The use of marijuana follows that of alcohol and tobacco. It is preceded by acceptance of a cluster of beliefs and values that often reflect disavowal of many standards upheld by adults. Involvement in a marijuana-using peer environment strongly predisposes to its use and is the best predictor (Becker, 1953; Goode, 1970). Participation in minor forms of deviant behaviors, such as those that also precede the use of hard liquor, is also an important precursor.

Antecedents of Adolescent Use of Marijuana

When use of marijuana first came under research scrutiny in the late 1960s, very few youths had experimented with illicit drugs. Much was made of the deviant status of use of marijuana and of the counter-cultural and rebellious meaning that came to be attached to using the drug (Suchman, 1968). Yet even today, when over 60 percent of all high school seniors have used marijuana, those youths who use marijuana are quite different from nonusers. The marijuana users in 1979 show the same patterns of disaffection from major institutions that characterized the users in 1967. The most recent data show that marijuana users perform more poorly in school, are less religious, have performed more delinquent acts, are in trouble with the law, have more traffic accidents, and use more illicit drugs than nonusers. Those persons who also use several illicit drugs show the highest involvement in deviant behaviors. There is a linear relationship with degree of involvement with illicit drugs, such that persons using marijuana exclusively are only quantitatively different from those who have also used harder drugs (Johnston et al., 1980b).

In two cross-sectional national samples of high school students, surveyed in 1974 and 1978, Jessor et al. have found that not only are the patterns of association between use of marijuana and deviant characteristics similar in both surveys, but also that the strength of the associations, as reflected in the sizes of the correlation coefficients, are almost identical. The very same conclusions derive from analyses based on five successive cohorts of high school seniors, sampled at yearly intervals in Monitoring the Future (Bachman et al., 1981).

Longitudinal studies of students aged 12-21 have done much to extend our understanding of the precursors of using various forms of drugs. Studies have been reviewed in detail by Kandel (1978a,b; 1980a; also see Appendix C) and document that many of the factors found to be associated with use of drugs at one point in time, such as low academic performance, crime, low self-esteem, depressive mood, rebelliousness, and other personality characteristics, precede the use of drugs (see in particular Mellinger et al., 1976; Jessor and Jessor, 1977; Johnston et al., 1978; Kandel, 1978a; Kandel et al., 1978b,c; Kaplan and Pokorny, 1978; Smith and Fogg, 1978; Wingard et al., 1979; Kaplan, 1980). Some of the predictive factors can be identified in childhood, such as aggressiveness with or without association with shyness (Kellam et al., 1980, in press) and rebelliousness (Smith and Fogg, 1978).

Other longitudinal studies also document that many of the factors found to be associated with use of drugs at one point in time, such as low academic performance, delinquency, low self-esteem, and depressive mood actually precede the use of drugs (O'Malley, 1975; Mellinger et al., 1976; Jessor and Jessor, 1977; Johnston et al., 1978; Kandel et al., 1978a; Kaplan and Pokorny, 1978; Wingard et al., 1979; Kaplan, 1980).

One study shows not only that certain behaviors predict use of marijuana, but also that drugs may aggravate or exaggerate certain behaviors. A cohort of high school students was followed at annual intervals throughout the four years of high school (Jessor and Jessor, 1977). During this time annual scores for various attributes were charted in four groups of students distinguished by differing drug histories: veteran users, who used drugs pre-high school; early initiates, who began relatively early in their high school career, i.e., between the first and second year of testing; late initiates, who began relatively late, i.e., between the second and the third year; and nonusers, who had not started to use marijuana at the last testing in the senior year of high school (Jessor and Jessor, 1977, 1978). These four groups of students differed on measures, such as general deviant behavior (a 12-item scale measuring frequency of involvement in stealing, fighting, property destruction, truancy, or other delinquent activities in the last year) or value on academic achievement (a five-item scale, measuring the value placed on the attainment of success in school work), at the beginning of the study. Scores predicted if and when students initiated use of marijuana. Those students already involved in use of drugs before high school scored highest on deviance and lowest on achievement motivation at initial testing and throughout subsequent retests. The scores of all groups of users converged over time so that all three groups increased in deviance scores and decreased in their achievement orientation over the four years. The sharpest changes in scores occurred in the year preceding the drug use.

Peer Influences

The most consistent and reproducible finding in drug research is the strong relationship between an individual's drug behavior and the concurrent use of drugs by his friends. The relationship is stronger when based on adolescents' perceptions of the friends' behavior than on the friends' self-reports (Goode, 1970; Johnson, 1973; Kandel, 1973; Goldstein, 1975; O'Donnell et al., 1976; Brook et al., 1977; Jessor and Jessor, 1977; Kandel et al., 1978a; Orcutt, 1978; Smart et al., 1978; Huba et al., 1979). On no other characteristic except age and sex is the similarity within adolescent friendship pairs as high as it is for use of marijuana (Kandel, 1978c). Such similarity results not only from socialization, the influence of one friend on the other, but also from a process of interpersonal selection (assortive pairing), in which adolescents with similar values and behavior seek each other out as friends. Longitudinal data on the formation and dissolution of friendships indicate that selection and socialization contribute about equally to the similarity in values and behaviors (Kandel, 1978d). Available data on sex differences in peer influence indicate that females are more susceptible than males to such influence (Jessor et al., 1973; Margulies et al., 1977). Susceptibility to peer influence is related to involvement in peer-related activities, e.g., dating or getting together with friends, and to degree of attachment to and reliance on peers rather than parents (Jessor and Jessor, 1978; Kandel et al., 1978a; Brook et al., 1980). Contact with other users increases the likelihood that the individual will have increased opportunities to get the drug. Peer-mediated approaches have been shown to be an effective vehicle for interventions to prevent smoking of tobacco in adolescents (Evans, 1977; McAlister, 1979). The powerful role of peer influence on the use of marijuana would seem to suggest that it would be also useful for preventive marijuana programs.

SUMMARY

There has been a steep rise in the use of marijuana and other illicit drugs in the past decade. So far it is primarily a youth phenomenon. Since 1971 there has been at least a doubling of lifetime experience with marijuana in every cohort in the 12- to 24-year age group. Of all psychoactive drugs investigated (including inhalants, hallucinogens, cocaine, heroin, stimulants, sedatives, and tranquilizers), marijuana is by far the most commonly used illicit drug. Legal drugs for adults, such as alcohol and tobacco, are the most widely used of all drugs among adolescents. Although substantially more students have ever used alcohol in their lifetime than have ever used marijuana, more high school seniors use marijuana on a "daily" basis (9 percent) than use alcohol that frequently (6 percent). "Daily" users report the use of marijuana in school, whereas daily use of alcohol tends to occur after school and on weekends.

Some trends in use of marijuana are apparent. The continuing dramatic rise in the use of marijuana has recently slowed. It is too early to tell whether this decrease will continue or is merely a pause in the rise. The overall prevalence of use of marijuana has remained at approximately 60 percent of high school seniors for the years 1978, 1979, and 1980. Between 1975 and 1978 there was an almost twofold increase in "daily" use of marijuana from 6 percent in 1975 to a peak rate of 11 percent in 1978. In 1980 the "daily" use rate of high school seniors dropped by 1.2 percentage points, or more than 10 percent. This may signal a reversal of the upward trend in "daily" use unless higher absenteeism and school drop-out of daily users are significant factors in the decline. Multiple sources suggest that out-of-school age mates are heavier users than those in school. Other trends have not slowed. There was a continuing rise in 1980 of the proportion of high school seniors who during the year had used some illicit drug other than marijuana, from 28 percent in 1979 to 30 percent in 1980.

Throughout the 1970s, as a correlate of continuing rise in prevalence rates, there was a trend toward younger ages of first use of all of these drugs. For marijuana this age trend continues but has slowed somewhat. In 1979, 23 percent of seniors who had used marijuana started their use in the eighth grade or below as compared to 25 percent in 1980.

"Daily" use of marijuana in high school and in early adult life is very high and merits special attention. Drawing on data from Monitoring the Future, characteristics of "daily" users were described. For high school seniors the rate of "daily" marijuana use in 1980 was 9.1 percent. Such users have very high involvement with other drugs and begin their use of drugs at very early ages. "Daily" users are predominantly urban although rates do not vary by geographical regions of the country, whereas use among white students is double that for blacks. "Daily" use is only slightly higher in disrupted or single parent homes than in nuclear families, and use is associated with poor school achievement, absenteeism, and dropout. Non-college-bound students are twice as likely to be "daily" users as were students planning to attend college. Religious commitment and self-ratings of strong belief in law-abiding behavior are associated with lower "daily" use rates. "Daily" users are involved in more automobile accidents and delinquency.

Post-high school "daily" user rates are lowest among full-time college students and those living in a college dormitory. "Daily" use among non-college students was not related to joblessness, employment, or military service. Single persons are twice as likely as married persons to be "daily" users. Among the married, those with children had very low rates of "daily" use. The "daily" use habit has a remarkable stability. By 4 years after high school, 85 percent of "daily" using seniors in the class of 1975 were still using marijuana, with 51 percent of them continuing to be "daily" users.

In these studies, students report reasons for using marijuana: to have a good time with friends, to get "high," to relieve boredom, to enhance the effects of other drugs, and to cope with stress. "Daily" users are deeply immersed in a drug-using circle of friends.

Some "daily" users have discontinued their habit. Reasons given for stopping use of marijuana are loss of interest in getting "high," concern about harmful physical or psychological effects, and concern about their loss of energy or ambition.

More is known about the antecedents of using marijuana than is known about the consequences of using marijuana (to be discussed further in the chapters that follow). Longitudinal studies have established that use of marijuana is preceded by acceptance of a cluster of beliefs and values that are favorable to use of marijuana and also by the adoption of deviant behaviors. The deviant psychosocial attributes of marijuana users that were described almost a decade ago, when use of marijuana was a rare event, are just as characteristic of marijuana users today, when 60 percent of all high school seniors report some experience with the use of marijuana. Daily users show the extremes of these deviant behaviors but less deeply involved users also exhibit some deviancy. Friendship patterns and peer influence play a uniquely powerful role in determining youthful marijuana use. Negative parental relationships do not appear to be associated as an antecedent to use of marijuana.

RECOMMENDATIONS FOR RESEARCH

Additional research needed includes (1) epidemiologic studies on patterns of use of drugs among young adolescents, including those who leave school, (2) longitudinal studies to investigate the antecedents and consequences of use of marijuana, and (3) studies of the effects of marijuana in combination with use of other drugs.

Because samples of high school seniors exclude youths most at risk for high marijuana involvement, namely adolescents not regularly attending the high school, additional cohort-sequential epidemiologic surveys beginning with prepubertal children are needed in order to follow development and behavior from early in life. An all-conclusive approach would be both a prospective (concurrent) cohort study and a retrospective case-control study of possible outcomes of and risk factors for marijuana use (this recommendation is described in detail in Chapter 6).

"Daily" users have been understudied and may have the most severe risk in terms of loss of learning potential, biological risk, and psychosocial handicap. Studies should be undertaken to predict who among the large numbers of young people who try marijuana are at risk of becoming "daily" users.

Research on the factors involved in cessation of the use of marijuana should also be carried out. Tobacco smoking is declining among youth (National Institute of Education, 1979). The reasons for this decline could be applicable to marijuana use and should be sought.

Studies should be undertaken to learn how peer influence can be reliably used to moderate or prevent marijuana use in young adolescents.

Properly planned longitudinal cohort studies should be conducted on both the behavioral and physiological antecedents and consequences of the use of marijuana. Detailed and continuing medical and psychosocial data are needed on the life careers of American adults who use marijuana "daily." Retrospective studies of middle-aged and elderly persons who have a history of chronic heavy use of marijuana would be systematically studied for medical and psychosocial attributes and for effects on job performance. These are especially needed for urban industrialized populations.

Little is known about the consequences of using marijuana in combination with other drugs. Inasmuch as the rates of use of other drugs are so high, this is of great salience. Interdisciplinary and collaborative efforts are crucial if the complexities of multiple drugs and intercorrelated behaviors are to be disentangled.

REFERENCES

Bachman, J.G., Johnston, L.D., and O'Malley, P.M. Smoking, drinking, and drug use among American high school students: Correlates and trends, 1975-1979. Am. J. Public Health 71:59-69, 1981.

Becker, S. Becoming a marihuana user. Am. J. Sociol. 54:235-242, 1953.

Brook, J.S., Lukoff, I.F., and Whiteman, M. Peer, family, and personality domains as related to adolescents' drug behavior. Psychol. Rep. 41:1095-102, 1977.

Brook, J.S., Lukoff, I.F. and Whiteman, M. Initiation into adolescent marihuana use. J. Gen. Psychol. 137:133-142, 1980.

Burt, M.R., Biegal, M.M., Carnes, Y., and Farley, E.C. Worldwide Survey of Nonmedical Drug Use and Alcohol Use Among Military Personnel: 1980. Bethesda, Md.: Burt Associates, Inc., 1980.

Cisin, I., Miller, J.D., and Harrell, A. Highlights from the National Survey on Drug Abuse: 1977. Washington, D.C.: U.S. Government Printing Office, 1978.

Evans, R.I., Hansen, W.B., and Mittlemark, M.B. Increasing the validity of self-reports of behavior in smoking in children investigation. J. Appl. Psychol. 62:521-523, 1977.

Fishburne, P.M., Abelson, H.I., and Cisin, I. National Survey on Drug Abuse: Main Findings: 1979. DHHS Publication No. (ADM) 80-976. WAshington, D.C.: U.S. Government Printing Office, 1980.

Gallup Opinion Index, pp. 1-11. Report No. 143. Marijuana in America, 1976.

Goldstein, J.W. Assessing the interpersonal determinants of adolescent drug use, pp. 47-52. In Lettieri, D.J. (ed.)

54

Predicting Adolescent Drug Abuse: A Review of Issues, Methods
and Correlates. DHEW Publication No.(ADM)76-299. Washington,
D.C.: U.S. Government Printing Office, 1975.

Goode, E. The Marijuana Smokers New York: Basic Books, Inc., 1970.

Hamburg, B.A., Kraemer, H.C., and Jahnke, W. A hierarchy of drug use
in adolescence: Behavioral and attitudinal correlates of
substantial drug use. Am. J. Psychiatry 132:1155-1163, 1975.

Huba, G..J., Wingard, J.A., and Bentler, P.M. Beginning adolescent
drug use and peer and adult interaction patterns. J. Consult.
Clin. Psychol. 47:265-276, 1979.

Jessor, R. and Jessor, S.L. Problem Behavior and Psychosocial
Development: A Longitudinal Study of Youth. New York: Academic
Press, 1977.

Jessor, R. and Jessor, S.L. Theory testing in longitudinal research
on marihuana use, pp. 41-71. In Kandel, D. (ed.) Longitudinal
Research on Drug Use: Empirical Findings and Methodological
Issues. Washington, D.C.: Hemisphere Publishing Corp., 1978.

Jessor, R., Jessor, S.L., and Finney, J. A social psychology of
marijuana use: Longitudinal studies of high school and college
youth. J. Pers. Soc. Psychol. 26:1-15, 1973.

Jessor, R., Donovan, J.E., and Widmer, K. Psychosocial Factors in
Adolescent Alcohol and Drug Use: The 1978 National Sample Study,
and the 1974-78 Panel Study. Final Report. Boulder, Colo.:
University of Colorado Institute of Behavioral Science, 1980.

Johnson, B.D. Marijuana Users and Drug Subcultures New York: John
Wiley, 1973.

Johnson, B.D. and Uppal, G.S. Marihuana and youth: A generation
gone to pot, pp. 81-108. In Scarpitti, F.R. and Datesman, S.K.
(eds.) Drugs and the Youth Culture. Beverly Hills, Calif.: Sage
Publications, 1980.

Johnston, L.D. The daily marijuana user. Paper presented at the
Meeting of the National Alcohol and Drug Coalition, Washington,
D.C., September 18, 1980.

Johnston, L.D. Frequent marijuana use: Correlates, possible
effects, and reasons for using and quitting. Paper presented at
a Conference on Treating the Marijuana Dependent Person,
sponsored by the American Council on Marijuana and Other
Psychoactive Drugs, Bethesda, Md., May 4, 1981.

Johnston, L.D., O'Malley, P. and Eveland, L. Drugs and delinquency:
A search for causal connections, pp. 137-156. In Kandel, D.B.
(ed.) Longitudinal Research on Drug Use: Empirical Findings and
Methodological Issues. Washington, D.C.: Hemisphere Publishing
Corporation, 1978.

Johnston, L.D., Bachman, J.G., and O'Malley, P.M. Drugs and the
Class of '78: Behaviors, Attitudes, and Recent National Trends
DHEW Publication No.(ADM)79-877. Washington, D.C.: U.S.
Government Printing Office, 1979a.

Johnston, L.D., Bachman, J.G., and O'Malley, P.M. 1979 Highlights.
Drugs and the Nation's High School Students. Five Year National
Trends. DHHS Publication No.(ADM)81-930. Washington, D.C.:
U.S. Government Printing Office, 1979b.

Johnston, L.D., Bachman, J.G., and O'Malley, P.M. Highlights from Student Drug Use in America, 1975-1980. DHHS Publication No. (ADM)81-1066. Washington, D.C.: U.S. Government Printing Office, 1980a.

Johnston, L.D., Bachman, J.G., and O'Malley, P.M. Monitoring the Future. Questionnaire Responses from the Nation's High School Seniors 1979 Ann Arbor: Survey Research Center, The University of Michigan, 1980b.

Kandel, D. Adolescent marihuana use: Role of parents and peers. Science 181:1067-1070, 1973.

Kandel, D. Reaching the hard-to-reach: Illicit drug use among high school absentees. Addict. Dis. 1:465-80, 1975a.

Kandel, D. Stages in adolescent involvement in drug use. Science 190:912-914, 1975b.

Kandel, D. and Faust, R. Sequence and stages in patterns of adolescent drug use. Arch. Gen. Psychiatry 32:923-932, 1975.

Kandel, D.B. (ed.) Longitudinal Research on Drug Use: Empirical Findings and Methodological Issues. Washington, D.C.: Hemisphere Publishing Corp., 1978a.

Kandel, D.B. Convergences in prospective longitudinal surveys of drug use in normal populations, pp. 3-38. In Kandel, D.B. (ed.) Longitudinal Research on Drug Use: Empirical Findings and Methodological Issues. Washington, D.C.: Hemisphere Publishing Corp., 1978b.

Kandel, D.B. Similarity in real-life adolescent friendship pairs. J. Pers. Soc. Psychol. 36:306-312, 1978c.

Kandel, D.B. Homophily, selection, and socialization in adolescent friendships. Am. J. Sociol. 84:427-436, 1978d.

Kandel, D.B. Drug and drinking behavior among youth. Ann. Rev. Sociol. 6:235-285, 1980.

Kandel, D., Kessler, R., and Margulies, R. Antecedents of adolescent initiation into stages of drug use: A developmental analysis, pp. 73-99. In Kandel, D.B. (ed.) Longitudinal Research on Drug Use: Empirical Findings and Methodological Issues. Washington, D.C.: Hemisphere Publishing Corp., 1978a.

Kandel, D.B., Margulies, R.Z., and Davies, M. Analytical strategies for studying transitions into developmental stages. Sociol. Educ. 51:162-176, 1978b.

Kandel, D.B., Kessler, R.C., and Margulies, R.Z. Antecedents of adolescent initiation into stages of drugs use: A developmental analysis. J. Youth and Adolescence 7:13-40, 1978c.

Kandel, D.B., Adler, I., and Sudit, M. The epidemiology of adolescent drug use in France and Israel. Am. J. Public Health 71:256-265, 1981.

Kaplan, H.B. Deviant Behavior in Defense of Self New York: Academic Press, 1980.

Kaplan, H.B. and Pokorny, A.D. Alcohol use and self-enhancement among adolescents: A conditional relationship, pp. 51-75. In Seixaz, F.A. (ed.) Currents in Alcoholism. Volume IV: Psychiatric, Psychological, Social and Epidemiological Studies. New York: Grunne and Stratton, 1978.

Kellam, S.G., Ensminger, M.E., and Simon, M.B. Mental health in first grade and teenage drug, alcohol and cigarette use. J. Drug Alcohol Dependence May:273-304, 1980.

Kellam, S., Simon, M., and Ensminger, M.E. Antecedents in first grade of teenage drug use and psychological well-being: A ten year community-wide prospective study. In Ricks, D. and Dohrenwend, B. (eds.) Origins of Psychopathology: Research and Public Policy. Cambridge University Press (in press).

Margulies, R.Z., Kessler, R.C., and Kandel, D.B. A longitudinal study of onset of drinking among high-school students. J. Stud. Alcohol 38:897-912, 1977.

McAlister, A.L. Tobacco, alcohol, and drug abuse: Onset and prevention, pp. 197-206. In Healthy People: The Surgeon General's Report on Health Promotion and Disease Prevention, Background Papers, 1979. DHEW(PHS) Publication No. 79-55071A. Washington, D.C.: U.S. Government Printing Office, 1979.

Mellinger, G.D., Somers, R.M., Davidson, S.T., and Manheimer, D.I. The amotivational syndrome and the college student. Ann. N.Y. Acad. Sci. 282:37-55, 1976.

Miller, J.D. and Cisin, I.H. Highlights from the National Survey on Drug Abuse: 1979. DHHS Publication No. (ADM)80-1032. Washington, D.C.: U.S. Government Printing Office, 1980.

National Institute of Education. Teenage Smoking: Immediate and Long Term Patterns. Washington, D.C.: U.S. Government Printing Office, 1979.

O'Donnell, J.A., Voss, H.L., Clayton, R.R., et al. Young Men and Drugs--A Nationwide Survey NIDA Research Monograph 5. DHEW Publication No. (ADM)76-311. Washington, D.C.: U.S. Government Printing Office, 1976.

O'Malley, P.M. Correlates and Consequences of Illicit Drug Use. Ph.D. Thesis. University of Michigan, Ann Arbor. 326 pp. 1975.

Orcutt, J.D. Normative definitions of intoxicated states: A test of several sociological theories. Soc. Probl. 25:385-396, 1978.

Rittenhouse, J.D. Learning Drug Use: From "Legal" Substance to Marijuana and Beyond. Paper presented at the American Psychological Association Annual Convention, Montreal, Canada, September 1980.

Robins, L.N. The Vietnam Drug User Returns. Final Report. Special Action Office Monograph Series A, No. 2. Washington, D.C.: U.S. Government Printing Office, 1974.

Smart, R.G., Gray, G., and Bennett, C. Predictors of drinking and signs of heavy drinking among high school students. Int. J. Addict. 13:1079-1094, 1978.

Smith, G.M. and Fogg, C.P. Psychological predictors of early use, late use, and nonuse of marihuana among teenage students. pp. 101-113. In Kandel, D.B. (ed.) Longitudinal Research on Drug Use: Empirical Findings and Methodological Issues Washington, D.C.: Hemisphere Publishing Corp., 1978.

Suchman, E.A. The "hang-loose" ethic and the spirit of drug use. J. Health Soc. Behav. 9:146-155, 1968.

Wingard, J.A., Huba, G.J., and Bentler, P.M. The relationship of personality structure to patterns of adolescent substance use. Multivariate Behav. Res. 14:131-143, 1979.

3

EFFECTS OF MARIJUANA ON THE RESPIRATORY AND CARDIOVASCULAR SYSTEMS

RESPIRATORY SYSTEM

Performance (Pulmonary Function)

The lungs are the natural target for the harmful effects of smoked materials. This is as true for marijuana as for tobacco. In both instances, smoke is drawn into the lungs where it can harm not only the cells that line the airways (trachea, nasopharynx, bronchi, and alveoli) and constitute the lung tissue, but also impair such cells as lung macrophages, which are part of the immune system. As a result, the smoke may inflict injury directly on parts of the system and also make the lungs vulnerable to agents that normally are held at bay by self-cleansing and self-protecting mechanisms.

Different effects would be expected from tobacco and marijuana smoking because of the striking differences in the way in which the two substances are smoked: marijuana smoke usually is drawn deeply into the lungs by one or a few deliberately deep breaths, whereas tobacco smoking is generally more automatic, repetitive, and variable in pattern. Moreover, because marijuana is a "street drug," it not only is inconsistent in its content but also is subject to contamination. Also, filters are not usually used by marijuana smokers, although water pipes are used occasionally. Consequently, under natural conditions it is difficult to judge dosage of active ingredients, to sort out the influence of contaminants, and to compare the consequences of marijuana and tobacco smoke.

Experience over the years with cigarette smoking has shown that continued exposure to tobacco smoke entails the risk of producing chronic bronchitis and/or carcinoma of the lung. But, although cannabis products have been smoked for centuries, remarkably little is recorded about their effects on the lungs. Whatever contemporary information exists is confounded by the fact that most marijuana smokers are also tobacco smokers.

In recent years, interest has heightened in the smoking of marijuana as a therapeutic measure. The inhalation route takes advantage of the large surface area afforded by the lungs for administering the effective constituents of marijuana. However, this practice entails the disadvantage of administering a therapeutic agent in a cloud of air pollutants.

In brief, our appraisal must assess the impact of chronic bronchial irritation and inflammation on the airways and gas-exchanging surfaces of the lungs.

Acute Effects

Marijuana affects the control of the breathing pattern in different ways depending upon the dose, the preparation, and its psychotropic effect on the consumer. One marijuana cigarette generally stimulates ventilation (air exchange between the lungs and the ambient air) in conjunction with an increase in the metabolic rate and a heightened response to carbon dioxide (CO_2) as a regulatory stimulant (Vachon et al., 1973; Zwillich et al., 1978). On the other hand, larger doses of smoked marijuana may depress the ventilation and responsiveness to the CO_2 stimulus (Weil et al., 1968; Bellville et al., 1975). The intravenous administration of Δ-9-THC in equivalent doses has much less of an effect either on the ventilation or on the effectiveness of CO_2 as a respiratory stimulant (Malit et al., 1975).

Much more consistent and predictable is the effect of marijuana on the airways. The inhalation of small amounts of marijuana smoke causes bronchial dilation in persons without demonstrable lung disease (Tashkin et al., 1973; Vachon et al., 1973). The bronchodilation is easily demonstrable; the inhalation of isoproterenol (1250 µg), a potent bronchodilator, caused less of an improvement in airways conductance than the peak effect observed after smoking 2 percent marijuana (Tashkin et al., 1973). Ingestion of Δ-9-THC is less effective than smoking marijuana in producing bronchodilation; the bronchodilator effects of smoked marijuana last as long as 60 minutes; that of ingested Δ-9-THC up to 6 hours. Aerosolized Δ-9-THC has a local irritating effect on the airways, which often overrides the bronchodilating effect to the point of making it unsuitable for therapeutic purposes (Tashkin et al., 1977a).

Except for bronchodilation, acute exposure to marijuana has little effect on breathing as measured by conventional pulmonary tests. Thus, in young marijuana smokers (21-30 years of age) who smoked at least four cigarettes per week and no tobacco for at least 6 months before, ventilatory mechanics and gas exchange were normal by conventional tests (Tashkin et al., 1976). In contrast, heavy marijuana smoking, i.e., at least 4 days per week for 6 to 8 weeks did cause mild airway obstruction (Tashkin et al., 1976).

Acute smoking of marijuana, as well as the ingestion of Δ-9-THC, also causes bronchodilation in individuals with mild to moderate asthma (Tashkin et al., 1974). Marijuana smoking or ingestion of Δ-9-THC also dilated airways in asthmatics in whom bronchoconstriction was deliberately provided either by exercise or by the inhalation of methacholine, a bronchoconstrictor (Shapiro et al., 1976a). The mechanism by which bronchodilation is effected is not clear, but does not involve stimulation of beta-adrenergic receptors or blockade of muscarinic receptors in airway smooth muscle (Shapiro et al., 1976a). Adding to the difficulties of interpretation are the psychotropic effects of marijuana: four of the individuals who had previously used cannabis could distinguish the marijuana cigarette from the placebo on the basis of the intoxicating experience afforded by the marijuana smoke. Although the four subjects without previous cannabis experience did not experience any central nervous system effects, they did note mild somnolence or light-headedness after marijuana use.

Among the experiments with induced asthma were some that employed the inhalation of cannabinoid-free marijuana smoke (Tashkin et al., 1975). The results indicate that the smoke of the marijuana cigarette does not prevent methacholine-induced bronchospasm (Tashkin et al., 1976). Smoking of marijuana did not aggravate or perpetuate bronchoconstriction in stable asthmatics, and it promptly reversed experimentally induced bronchospasm (Tashkin et al., 1978). Addition of Δ-9-THC to placebo smoke caused a prompt, complete, and sustained reversal of methacholine-induced bronchospasm. Although ingestion of Δ-9-THC in a sesame oil vehicle has produced bronchodilation in asthmatic patients, less dilation was noted than after smaller doses of Δ-9-THC delivered by smoking (Tashkin et al., 1974).

Although it appears that the mechanism of Δ-9-THC-induced bronchial dilation is mediated by the autonomic nervous system, the process of dilation is not understood (Gill and Paton, 1970; Cavero et al., 1972; Shapiro et al., 1973).

Subacute Effects

Pulmonary function tests in 28 healthy young experienced cannabis users before and after a 47-59-day period of heavier than customary marijuana usage (group daily average of 5.2 cigarettes, with a daily mean range of 1.7 to 10 cigarettes per subject) disclosed the development of mild but significant decreases in specific airway conductance and forced expiratory flow as well as in diffusing capacity (Tashkin et al., 1976). Cessation, by reduction in smoking, gradually restored the tests toward normal. The clinical significance of these abnormalities is uncertain. The marijuana smoked and the impairment in pulmonary function, coupled with the observation that reversibility of function was incomplete 1 week after marijuana smoking had stopped, suggests that heavy marijuana smoking over a much longer period could lead to clinically significant and less readily reversible impairment of pulmonary function.

Chronic Effects

A study of 31 American soldiers stationed in West Germany who smoked large quantities of hashish (100 grams or more per month for periods of 6 to 15 months) found their ailments to be principally respiratory, including bronchitis, sinusitis, asthma, and rhinopharyngitis (inflammation of the nasopharynx) (Tennant et al., 1971). In one-third of the soldiers, sputum-producing coughs, difficulty in breathing, and wheezing followed 3 to 4 months of regular use of hashish. However, they had a normal chest radiograph and normal sputum. Antibiotics failed to relieve the symptoms. The symptomatic patients could not work and four required hospitalization. An unspecified decrease in hashish consumption improved their symptoms.

Pulmonary function tests in these individuals showed mild airway obstruction after 3 days of lessened hashish intake. Moreover, the response of these individuals to isoproterenol suggested that reversible bronchospasm and/or the accumulation of fluid in the bronchi was involved in the pathogenesis of the airway obstruction. Patch and serological tests failed to implicate allergy as a cause of the upper respiratory symptoms and signs.

In Jamaica (Hall, 1975), where marijuana usage is heavy, chronic bronchitis is frequent. However, marijuana smoking is usually associated with tobacco smoking, which confounds interpretation of the effects of marijuana alone. Adding to the uncertainty about the effects of marijuana as a cause of chronic regulatory abnormalities are two other studies, one in Jamaica (Rubin and Comitas, 1975) and the other in Costa Rica (Hernandez-Bolanos et al., 1976), which failed to find any difference in the prevalence of chronic respiratory disease between smokers and nonsmokers of marijuana. These results cannot be accepted as conclusive, because in each study the number of marijuana smokers was small, the subjects were not randomly selected, and the use of tobacco was not taken into account.

Much more convincing is a recent study (Tashkin et al., 1980) of 74 persons who smoked marijuana for 2 to 5 years, typically as frequently as several times per day, 3 to 6 days per week. Care was taken to obtain proper control groups. The results indicated that habitual smoking of marijuana causes a mild but significant increase in resistance to airflow in the large airways without an appreciable effect on conventional tests.

Another study was of 200 American soldiers stationed in West Germany who voluntarily sought medical attention for such respiratory symptoms as pharyngitis, sinusitis, bronchitis, and asthma related to chronic heavy hashish smoking (Henderson et al., 1972). Analysis of the hashish available and in use in the locale of this study showed concentrations of 5 to 10 percent Δ-9-THC. Two to 3 percent of samples were contaminated with cocaine, opium, morphine, spices, or feces. Two aspects of hashish smoking are relevant to the question of lung injury produced by hashish: 1) hashish is usually smoked in a pipe (occasionally in a water pipe), although it is occasionally eaten, drunk as a tea, or rolled into a cigarette and smoked, and 2) hashish smoke generally is regarded by users as burning much hotter than tobacco smoke.

Soldiers with pharyngitis usually smoked less than 25 grams of hashish monthly; those with bronchitis and asthma consumed more than 50 grams per month. The common complaint of sore throat in these heavy hashish smokers occurred most often in those who smoked hashish in a pipe without a screen or cotton filter; in them, the roof of the mouth and the back of the throat were inflamed. Persistent rhinitis (inflammation of the nasal mucous membranes) was present in 26 patients. As a rule, allergy could not be implicated in the nasopharyngeal manifestations. Treatment with antibiotics, decongestants, and phenylephrine (a vasoconstrictor) relieved the symptoms, but they recurred in those who continued smoking hashish.

Twenty high-dose hashish smokers (more than 50 grams/month) had chronic bronchitis as manifested by a chronic sputum-producing cough, shortness of breath, and decreased exercise tolerance. On physical examination, abnormal respiratory sounds--rhonchi, wheezes, and rales--were present. Chest radiographs were consistently normal, but pulmonary function was abnormal; the vital capacity (the maximum volume of gas taken in) was 15 to 40 percent below normal. In six of these subjects who smoked 50 or more grams per month, biopsy of bronchial mucosa revealed changes that resembled the abnormalities that occur in older heavy smokers of tobacco (Auerbach et al., 1961). The biopsies also turned up atypical cells not found in tobacco smokers.

The study of a respiratory disease in hashish or marijuana smokers is difficult because the great majority also smoke tobacco cigarettes. Also, the illegality of marijuana smoking prevents people from volunteering information and cooperating in experimental studies. Baseline physiological or clinical studies are difficult, because the subject is not identified until he seeks medical help.

Rats (Fleischman et al., 1979) and dogs (Roy et al., 1976) have been exposed experimentally to marijuana smoke over long periods (1 year and 900 days, respectively) to determine its morphological effects on the lungs. At autopsy, the animals demonstrated damage of the airways and also of the lung substance. However, it is difficult to relate the results of these animal experiments, in which the artificial pattern of smoking differed markedly from that of the human smoker, to the effects that chronic marijuana smoking might elicit in man.

Defense Mechanisms (Alveolar Macrophages)

Little is known about the effects of marijuana on the defense mechanisms of the lungs. Although some observations have been made on the alveolar macrophage, an important element in this system, the results have been inconsistent. For example, some studies of the rat lung found that macrophages obtained by washing out the lung and exposing them to marijuana smoke manifested a depression in bactericidal activity (Huber et al., 1975, 1979a,b, 1980). On the other hand, another report failed to disclose a significant effect, not only of marijuana, but also of tobacco smoke on the bactericidal activity of macrophages (Drath et al., 1979). Finally, others have found that alveolar macrophages differ slightly in their morphological responses to tobacco and to marijuana smoke. The significance of these differences, especially in terms of their long-term effect on pulmonary defense mechanisms, remains to be defined.

Explants of lung have also been examined after exposure in culture to marijuana smoke (Leuchtenberger et al., 1973a,b; Leuchtenberger and Leuchtenberger, 1976). Striking changes have been observed in the appearance and growth characteristics of exposed cells.

Carcinoma of the Lung

The effect of marijuana as a carcinogen for lung, airways, and upper respiratory organs has not been systematically explored. Evaluating the carcinogenicity of marijuana is difficult, because most marijuana smokers also are tobacco cigarette smokers and because such carcinogenicity could have a long period of latency; studies of tobacco carcinogenesis indicate that 20 to 30 years of exposure must occur before tumors appear in the lung. It is understandable that information concerning the carcinogenic properties of marijuana are not yet available, particularly in the United States, where the agent has come into extensive use only during the past two decades. An important problem in evaluating carcinogenicity is the fact that the leaf is used by igniting it and the inhaled products of its combustion may be carcinogenic, as in the case of tobacco products. Even if it proved to be carcinogenic, the question would still remain as to what constituent in marijuana smoke was at fault.

The potency of a substance as a mutagen (ability to change genetic material) can provide a clue as to its possible role as a carcinogen. Induction of genetic mutations by a substance in test strains of bacteria correlates with induction of tumors in test animals. Fractions from extracts of marijuana smoke particulates ("tar") have been found to produce dose-related mutations in four out of five test strains of bacteria (Busch et al., 1979; Seid and Wei, 1979; Wehner et al., 1980). By itself, Δ-9-THC was not active as a mutagen in bacterial strains (Glatt et al., 1979) or in mammalian test systems (van Went, 1978).

The extent to which marijuana smoke differs from tobacco smoke is discussed in detail in Chapter 1. In general, except for the presence of cannabinoids in one and tobacco alkaloids (nicotine) in the other, the combustion products of tobacco and marijuana are qualitatively similar. On occasion, however, differences that may be meaningful have been found. For example, one study (Hoffmann et al., 1975) reports that tobacco smoke contains more isoprene and volatile phenols, whereas marijuana smoke contains about 50 percent more carcinogenic hydrocarbons.

Tumorigenicity of marijuana and tobacco smoke condensates on mouse skin have been reported. In mice painted three times weekly with a tar suspension of smoke condensate, survival at 74 weeks was better in the marijuana group than in the tobacco group. Six of 100 mice painted with marijuana condensate developed skin tumors, all of which were benign, whereas 14 of 100 in the tobacco condensate group developed tumors, two of them malignant (Hoffman et al., 1975).

Because marijuana smoke has adverse actions similar to tobacco smoke on cell function in the respiratory and cardiovascular systems, it has been proposed that marijuana smoke, rather than only the cannabinoid, should be used to obtain information about effects on cell injury and response (Leuchtenberger and Leuchtenberger, 1971). Exposure of human lung cells in culture to freshly generated marijuana smoke for up to 2 months resulted in increased mitotic indices, stimulation of DNA synthesis, and an increase in the population of cells with four times the DNA content of control cells or those exposed to tobacco smoke (Leuchtenberger et al., 1973a,b). Long-term exposure of hamster lung cells to the smoke of either marijuana or tobacco led to abnormal proliferation and malignant transformation within 3 to 6 months of exposure (Leuchtenberger and Leuchtenberger, 1976). Since malignant transformation was also noted in unexposed lung cells after 12-24 months of culture, it appears that the smoke of marijuana or tobacco accelerates, rather than initiates, the malignant change.

Although no instance of human lung carcinoma attributable solely to marijuana smoking has yet been reported, abnormalities suggestive of cancerous lesions have been recorded. For example, in several of the U.S. servicemen who smoked 50 grams of hashish or more per month and developed upper respiratory disorders, mucosal biopsy showed extensive cellular abnormalities, including loss of cilia, proliferation of basal epithelial cells, and atypical cells (Tennant et al., 1971; Henderson et al., 1972). Comparison of 30 American hashish smokers (25-150 grams/month for 3-24 months; 23 also smoked tobacco and 7 did not), 3 tobacco smokers (1.6 packs/day for 11.3 years) who did not smoke marijuana and 3 nonsmokers of tobacco or hashish, indicated exposure to combined marijuana and tobacco smoke produced more harmful effects than that produced by either substance alone (Tennant et al., 1980). In the hashish smokers who did not smoke tobacco, abnormalities in the tracheal biopsies were no more frequent or severe than in those persons who smoked only tobacco.

Exception has been taken to the idea of an additive effect of tobacco and hashish smoke. A Greek study that compared chronic hashish and tobacco users with tobacco smoking controls found that although the hashish smokers had considerably more throat irritation and cough, the prevalence of bronchitis in both groups was about the same (Boulougouris et al., 1976); no biopsies were taken. The differences between the Greek and American studies may reflect differences between the two populations: The American study, done in Germany, favored inclusion of men with severe respiratory disturbances (Tennant et al., 1980), whereas the Greek study (Boulougouris et al., 1976) appears to have included persons with less severe illness.

The finding of known carcinogens in marijuana smoke and the presence of epithelial abnormalities known to be the precursors of lung cancer in heavy smokers of tobacco suggest the possible development of lung cancer in chronic, heavy users of marijuana and/or hashish after a prolonged period of use, especially if they are also smokers of tobacco. However, evidence to support this hypothesis is not available. Because marijuana smoking is an ancient custom in Asia and the Middle East, lung cancer would be expected to be more prevalent in these parts of the world if a causal relationship did exist. Unfortunately, no reliable data have been gathered to settle this question. Heavy smoking of marijuana, in quantities comparable to that of tobacco, has been relatively uncommon in the United States. Therefore, the contribution of marijuana smoking to the incidence of primary lung cancer cannot yet be answered with any authoritative data.

Summary: Respiratory System

Lung Function and Defense Mechanisms

The most important question about the effects of marijuana on the health of the respiratory system is whether acute or chronic marijuana smoking cause detectable structural or functional impairment of the lungs. Mild but measurable airway obstruction, affecting both large and small airways, can be shown to exist after 6 to 8 weeks of smoking marijuana daily, averaging five marijuana cigarettes a day; this decrement in function is reversible, but does not return to normal within one week of abstaining from smoking.

In persons with histories of heavy smoking, particularly of hashish, chronic inflammatory changes are seen in the bronchi and uvula, often in association with chronic sinusitis. These manifestations of upper respiratory disturbance have been described in individuals with histories of marijuana smoking usually in excess of 3 years and are reversible when marijuana smoking is stopped.

Acute exposure of alveolar macrophages _in vitro_ to marijuana smoke causes a reduction in phagocytic activity, a cell defense mechanism. The agents responsible for this change in macrophage function are in the vapor phase of marijuana smoke and are not related to the presence of Δ-9-THC. Also, lung explants exposed to marijuana smoke _in vitro_ show changes in the chromosomal structure of nuclei.

There is as yet no information about the effects of prolonged smoking of marijuana, that is, beyond 5 years. Although some populations have been examined for the effects of chronic marijuana smoking, controlled studies are sparse and populations exposed to marijuana smoke only--without exposure to tobacco--apparently are not available. Particularly conspicuous is the lack of information about the effect of chronic marijuana smoking begun in late childhood or adolescence and continued to adulthood. Such studies would require morphological examination of biopsy material from the bronchi and respiratory passages to determine the presence of structural changes that indicate the development of chronic bronchitis and/or lung cancer. Morphological changes associated with smoking marijuana could be compared with the morphological abnormalities associated with chronic tobacco smoking.

The acute response to inhalation of marijuana is an appreciable bronchodilation, both in normal subjects and in individuals with bronchial asthma. However, the bronchodilator effects of marijuana are a response to acute exposure; chronic exposure usually evokes bronchoconstriction.

With respect to therapeutic application, the effects of smoking marijuana in producing bronchial dilatation do not exceed those that follow the inhalation of beta-agonist drugs. Moreover, the doses required for bronchodilatation usually elicit the psychotropic effects of marijuana and may be associated with changes in the structure of bronchial and parenchymal lung cells, the significance of which remains to be assessed. For these reasons therapeutic usefulness as a bronchodilator drug is open to serious question (see Chapter 7).

Carcinoma of the Lung

One of the great uncertainties about marijuana smoking is its neoplastic potential. No reliable data are available concerning the incidence of carcinoma of the lungs and upper respiratory passages in long-term users of cannabis.

But a variety of experimental studies has sounded the alert that marijuana smoking--just as tobacco smoking--may be carcinogenic and that a combination of tobacco and marijuana smoke may have greater neoplastic potential than either one alone. Although the experimental observations have raised the suspicion, long-term observations on human subjects--and possibly on smoking animals--will be necessary to settle the issue.

Recommendations for Research

Lung Function and Defense Mechanisms

With respect to the performance and defenses of the lungs, these studies would be informative:

* the physiological, biochemical, and morphological interactions of combined exposures of the respiratory tract to tobacco and marijuana smoke;
* the interactions of cannabis and alcohol on the function of the respiratory tract;
* the long-term effects, i.e., 10 to 30 years, of exposure of the respiratory tract to frequent use of cannabis in the absence and pressure of exposure to tobacco smoke (for this purpose, large-scale epidemiological studies may be required);
* the physiological effects and clinical consequences of exposure of alveolar macrophages and other lung cells to long-term exposure to marijuana smoke;
* the immunologic effects of marijuana smoke exposure on cells and on the entire body.

Carcinoma of the Lung

With respect to carcinoma of the lung, these studies seem essential:

- an epidemiological survey to determine over the next 20 to 30 years if there will be an increased incidence of primary lung, laryngeal, oropharyngeal, esophageal, nasal, or sinus cancer in chronic marijuana smokers;
- epidemiologic and pathological studies in humans and experimental studies in animals to evaluate the carcinogenic potential of chronic marijuana smoking on the lung, larynx, oropharynx, nasal, and sinus epithelium.

CARDIOVASCULAR SYSTEM

Normal Heart and Circulation

Heart (Direct Effects)

With respect to the heart and circulation, the most evident effect in human beings of smoking marijuana, or of ingesting the active ingredient (Δ-9-THC), is a brisk increase in heart rate (tachycardia). Although this is not threatening to the normal heart, the rapid heart action can be harmful to the heart in which the circulation is compromised by atherosclerosis or is on the verge of failing.

The responses of the cardiovascular system to acute exposure to marijuana differ between human beings and most other mammals in that the human subject typically responds with an increase in heart rate (Bright et al., 1971; Beaconsfield et al., 1972; Perez-Reyes et al., 1973), whereas most mammals show a slowing in rate (bradycardia) (Cavero et al., 1973; Graham and Li, 1973; Rosenkrantz and Braude, 1974; Vollmer et al., 1974; Adams et al., 1976; Hardman and Hosko, 1976; Kawasaki et al., 1980). Human blood pressure usually increases moderately on acute administration of Δ-9-THC, but in monkeys and dogs acute administration is followed by a decrease in systemic arterial pressure. Typical effects on heart rate and blood pressure have been attributed to altered autonomic function (Loewe, 1944; Joachimoglu, 1965; Ames, 1968; Gill and Paton, 1970).

Effects on the cardiovascular system are to some extent a function of dose, route of administration, and duration of exposure. Tolerance to some of the cardiovascular effects in human beings develops with chronic use (Benowitz and Jones, 1975, 1977a,b; Nowlan and Cohen, 1977), but continued use does not result in any persistent alteration in cardiovascular function after cessation of exposure (Dornbush and Kokkevi, 1976).

Effects on Heart Rate   In healthy young adults, acute administration of marijuana by smoking (10 mg total dose) causes a prompt increase in heart rate (increasing by up to 90 beats/minute) for about 1 hour.

The change in heart rate caused by Δ-9-THC appears to result from
alterations in both sympathetic and parasympathetic efferent activity
to the normal cardiac pacemaker (Beaconsfield et al., 1972; Martz et
al., 1972; Sulkowski et al., 1977). The results of studies designed
to determine whether beta-adrenergic stimulation is responsible for
the tachycardia have not been consistent: In one series of reports,
prior administration of propranolol,* in a dose sufficient to block
the heart's beta-adrenergic receptors, prevented the increase in
heart rate (Bright et al., 1971; Beaconsfield et al., 1972;
Perez-Reyes et al., 1973), whereas in other reports, propranolol
failed to block the marijuana-induced tachycardia (Kanakis et al.,
1976; Tashkin et al., 1978). Although part of the discrepancy may be
attributable to differences in dosages, not all of it can be
rationalized this way, leaving an unexplained disparity.

Hemodynamic Effects   Effects of marijuana on blood pressure and
cardiac output, as mentioned above, are a function of the nature of
exposure (acute or chronic), of the dose, and of the body position;
also, there are differences among human beings and a number of
mammalian species. In human beings lying supine, acute exposure to
Δ-9-THC typically causes a modest increase in blood pressure,
although in some instances no significant change in pressure has been
observed (Beaconsfield et al., 1972; Kanakis et al., 1976; Benowitz
et al., 1979). On assuming the upright posture, blood pressure may
drop considerably. Cardiac output, in the supine position following
an injection of Δ-9-THC, has been found to increase by as much as
30 percent (Malit et al., 1975; Tashkin et al., 1977b). The increase
in cardiac output in the face of only a modest increase in blood
pressure clearly results in a substantial decrease in peripheral
vascular resistance. The change in resistance varies among the
different vascular beds, being greatest in the vessels to the
skeletal muscles.

Chronic administration of quite large oral doses of Δ-9-THC
exerts different effects (than the acute) on the circulation
(Bernstein et al., 1974; Benowitz and Jones, 1975; Benowitz et al.,
1979). Systolic and diastolic pressure usually fall slightly, but
these changes are not always sustained. As the blood pressure falls,
the heart rate slows from the high levels caused by initial marijuana
administration. The decrease in blood pressure can be accentuated if
the subject assumes an upright posture. The extent to which it drops
appears to be a reciprocal function of the extent to which plasma
volume has increased.

Effects on Heart Muscle   Data about changes in human left
ventricular function caused by marijuana are not entirely convincing
because most studies have relied on noninvasive measurements and

---

*Propranolol is an agent that blocks beta-adrenergic neurotransmitters
and is used in treatment of cardiac arrhythmias.

because it has not been possible to control separately the several variables that modify left ventricular function and are changed by administration of Δ-9-THC. Changes in heart rate, afterload (systemic vascular resistance, blood pressure), or preload (plasma volume, venous return) individually can cause changes in heart size and ventricular performance. In spite of these limitations, conclusions can be drawn from the observations on human beings. Definitive animal studies of Δ-9-THC effects on ventricular performance have not been done.

Indices of cardiac performance usually improve after marijuana or Δ-9-THC. Almost invariably this improvement can be attributed to the increase in heart rate (Gash et al., 1978). The acute administration of Δ-9-THC (25 μg/kg intravenously) to healthy young males elicits, in association with the increase in heart rate, changes in the ventricular contraction periods (an increase in ejection time and shortening of the preinjection period), while systemic arterial pressure is unaffected (Weiss et al., 1972; Kanakis et al., 1976). Beta-adrenergic blockade by propranolol is followed by less striking changes in the contraction time intervals. Another study of 17 subjects who smoked two to three cigarettes (20 mg Δ-9-THC per cigarette) found cardiac output increased by 28 percent and heart rate by 30 percent, in conjunction with a slight decrease in stroke volume, which affects pulse pressure (Tashkin et al., 1977b).

Autonomic Nervous System

Marijuana could influence autonomic function in several ways: (1) by changing the sensitivity of reflexes that influence and control cardiovascular function; this effect could result either from changes in the processing of nerve impulses in the central nervous system or autonomic ganglia (a group of nerve cells outside the central nervous system), from changes in the liberation or metabolism of transmitters at the autonomic nerve terminals, or from changes in the sensitivity of the pre- or postjunctional receptors; (2) by a change in the levels of neurotransmitters, the catecholamines (norepinephrine, epinephrine) in the blood as a result of actions on the adrenal medulla, which secretes these neurotransmitters; activation of the adrenals could be a direct effect or by reflexes or by a central action of Δ-9-THC; and (3) by exerting effects on dopamine activity (an intermediate product in the synthesis of norepinephrine) either in the central nervous system or periphery.

Unfortunately, it is unclear how the effects of Δ-9-THC are exerted on the autonomic nervous system (Truitt and Anderson, 1971; Beaconsfield et al., 1972; Weiss et al., 1972; Englert et al., 1973; Ho et al., 1973; Howes and Osgood, 1974; Ho and Johnson, 1976; Huot, 1976; Benowitz and Jones, 1977a,b; Gash et al., 1978; Stefanis, 1978). The data are insufficient to determine if the effects come by way of the central nervous system, or by peripheral neural structures, or by the adrenal medulla. It is also difficult to assess the role of reflex adjustments in the heart and systemic circulation. Finally, other possibilities, such as desensitization or blockade of peripheral adrenergic receptors, have not been examined.

Although the data on human beings are not adequate to determine how marijuana influences autonomic function, evidence that it does has been obtained. For example, Δ-9-THC appears to reduce a number of autonomic reflexes: After marijuana, the typical changes in heart rate and blood pressure elicited by the Valsalva maneuver (a forced exhalation effort against the closed glottis) are decreased, and so are the reflex circulatory responses to immersion of the hand in cold water (Beaconsfield et al., 1972; Benowitz et al., 1979). However, during chronic administration of Δ-9-THC, no change occurs in the reflex decrease in heart rate caused by infusion of a dose of the vasoconstrictor phenylephrine sufficient to increase the blood pressure (Benowitz and Jones, 1975; Benowitz et al., 1979).

Exercise

Acute exposure to Δ-9-THC modifies exercise performance by human beings. Smoking (20 mg of Δ-9-THC) decreased the duration of exercise but caused no change in any cardiopulmonary parameter at any work load except for heart rate, which increased (Shapiro et al., 1976b).

Other Effects (Plasma Volume, Sodium Retention)

Acute administration of Δ-9-THC would not be expected to have prominent effects on sodium balance or plasma volume. Chronic administration, on the other hand, has distinct effects. With chronic ingestion of large doses of Δ-9-THC there is a consistent gain in body weight and plasma volume, the latter caused by sodium retention (Benowitz and Jones, 1975, 1977a,b). The change in plasma volume seems to be causally related to the decrease in orthostatic hypotension during chronic exposure. The mechanisms responsible for the retention of salt and water have not been explored and may include changes in renal perfusion, inhibition of prostaglandin (a substance that affects blood pressure) synthesis by Δ-9-THC (Burstein and Raz, 1972; Howes and Osgood, 1976), or some modification in pituitary-adrenal function (Birmingham and Bartova, 1976).

Abnormal Heart and Circulation

Although smoking marijuana or the introduction of Δ-9-THC into the body is apparently without deleterious effect on the normal heart and circulation, the possibility is great that the abnormal heart and circulation will not be as tolerant of an agent that speeds up the heart, sometimes unpredictably raises or drops the blood pressure, and modifies the activities of the autonomic nervous system. Therefore, it is pertinent to examine the prospects that marijuana (or Δ-9-THC) may be harmful in individuals with coronary heart disease, cerebrovascular disease, hypertension, and heart failure. Moreover, it may be important to determine if Δ-9-THC interacts in its effects on the abnormal heart or circulation with other agents that are being administered for therapeutic purposes.

Coronary Heart Disease

Data on this topic are sparse, presumably because of the relatively short time that marijuana has been available in this country. Those who have smoked marijuana are just entering the age when coronary atherosclerosis is common. However, it has been shown both in normal individuals and in individuals with coronary artery disease that the acute administration of Δ-9-THC by smoking or injection can cause changes in the electrocardiogram (ECG) (Johnson and Domino, 1971; Beaconsfield et al., 1972; Kochar and Hosko, 1973). Premature beats have also been noted. The reasons for the changes are unclear. Also not understood is the contribution of the increase in heart rate itself to the ECG changes and to the premature beats.

In some patients with coronary artery disease, increased catecholamines can induce arrhythmias. It seems likely that in such patients Δ-9-THC could have the same effect. Also, in patients with coronary artery disease a large increase in heart rate can induce angina (pain) and even ischemic damage from insufficient oxygen as a result of an obstructed blood vessel. If Δ-9-THC were to increase heart rate markedly in such patients, and at the same time increase the need for cardiac perfusion because of the increased cardiac work and because of the intensified effect of catecholamines on the heart, it seems reasonable that there could be induction of angina and potentially precipitation of ischemic damage. Furthermore, if Δ-9-THC dulled the appreciation of pain and the appropriate responses to pain, the patient might not take suitable measure to relieve the angina, thereby increasing the risk of damage or arrhythmias.

A decrease in oxygen-carrying capacity of blood because of formation of carboxyhemoglobin could also be troublesome. Exercise tolerance has been reported to decrease in individuals with angina after smoking marijuana; this decrease is in contrast to the unaffected exercise tolerance after smoking a placebo marijuana cigarette (Aronow and Cassidy, 1974). Oral ingestion of Δ-9-THC or smoking marijuana apparently can cause marked hypertension in association with an increase in systemic vascular resistance (Benowitz et al., 1979), which would place the heart with coronary artery disease at risk of damage.

These observations concur in indicating that marijuana and Δ-9-THC increase the work of the heart, often in many ways. The conclusion seems inescapable that this increased work, coupled with stimulation by catecholamines, may tax the heart to the point of clinical hazard.

Cerebrovascular Disease

There are few, if any, indications that Δ-9-THC has direct effects on the cerebral circulation that would be important in patients with cerebrovascular disease. In the occasional patient who develops hypertension after smoking, there would be an increased risk of a cerebral vascular accident (stroke). Also, because Δ-9-THC administered after atropine can cause marked increases in blood pressure, this combination would place the patient with cerebrovascular disease at risk, as would smoking after ingestion of other muscarinic blockers. In some patients, postural hypotension could be a problem, not only for persons with abnormal cerebral circulations, but also with abnormal coronary circulations.

Hypertension

The factors that act to intensify angina would be of importance in hypertensive patients. Although data are lacking on the magnitude of change in blood pressure caused by Δ-9-THC in hypertensives, it seems reasonable to assume that hypertensives smoking marijuana might have a greater increase in blood pressure than normals do. The increase in plasma volume and sodium retention that are associated with chronic exposure to Δ-9-THC could increase blood pressure in hypertensives and the mechanisms responsible for these changes very likely would interfere with the action of a number of antihypertensive medications.

Heart Failure

Because marijuana can cause tachycardia, a decrease in systemic vascular resistance (required for increased cardiac output to sustain blood pressure) and salt and water retention might place patients with severe heart failure at a disadvantage by exposure to Δ-9-THC. Data on such patients are lacking. In older patients treated by Δ-9-THC or who have smoked marijuana for glaucoma or cancer, orthostatic hypotension has been both disabling and a threat of cardiovascular complications (Merritt et al., 1980). However, tolerance to orthostatic hypotension seems to develop during continued intake of Δ-9-THC or continued smoking of marijuana. Dehydration, as during vomiting or diuretic therapy, predisposes to the orthostatic hypotensive effects and resists the development of tolerance because it prevents expansion of blood volume.

Interactions with Cardioactive Drugs

Few studies evaluate interactions between Δ-9-THC and other drugs that act directly or indirectly on the heart. Propranolol usually attenuates the increase in heart rate caused by Δ-9-THC. Atropine can greatly potentiate the ability of Δ-9-THC to increase systemic arterial pressure (Benowitz and Jones, 1977a,b). A number of possible interactions can be imagined. If a patient were taking a drug that blocked uptake of catecholamines by nerve terminals, then those effects of Δ-9-THC that are mediated by catecholamines would be intensified. Because a great many psychotropic and antihypertensive drugs modify metabolism of neurotransmitters in the central nervous system and periphery, a wide variety of interactions with Δ-9-THC seems possible.

Summary: Cardiovascular System

The smoking of marijuana causes changes in the heart and circulation that are characteristic of stress. But there is no evidence to indicate that it exerts a permanently deleterious effect on the normal cardiovascular system. Neither is there convincing evidence that marijuana would be of particular benefit in treating any of the major forms of cardiovascular disease.

The situation is quite different for those with an abnormal heart or circulation. Evidence abounds that marijuana increases the work of the heart, usually by increasing heart rate, and in some persons by increasing blood pressure. This increase in workload poses a threat to patients with hypertension, cerebrovascular disease, and coronary atherosclerosis. The magnitude and incidence of the threat remains to be determined because marijuana smoking has largely been confined to younger adults who are only now entering the age of serious complications of atherosclerosis on the heart, brain, and peripheral vessels.

Marijuana also can cause postural hypotension. This drop in blood pressure could be hazardous in those individuals with compromised blood flow to the heart or brain, especially if they are volume-depleted (dehydrated) or if other drugs have impaired reflex control of their blood vessels.

Marijuana appears to intensify the effects of the sympathetic nervous system on the heart, an undesirable consequence in patients with coronary artery disease and in those susceptible to arrhythmias. Many of the undesirable effects of marijuana on the cardiovascular system seem to become less severe following chronic exposure. Whether the relative paucity of reports of the ill-effects of marijuana on the abnormal cardiovascular system is a consequence of adaptation to chronic usage or to lack of exposure to marijuana of a population that is sufficiently advanced in years to be susceptible to its untoward effects remains to be determined.

Recommendations for Research

Additional studies are needed both (1) to provide information on the mechanisms responsible for the observed effects of marijuana on the cardiovascular system and (2) to provide new data on the effects of marijuana in patients with known forms of cardiovascular disease.

· The manner in which Δ-9-THC acts on the heart to change the rate and force of contraction needs clarification. Direct effects on the heart are not likely to differ among species, and thus experiments can be planned for a "standard" heart preparation.

· Direct effects on electrical activity, which might relate to reports of changes in electrical activity and production of premature impulses as well as changes in sinus rate, should be evaluated with standard methods and standard preparations.

· Direct effects of Δ-9-THC on vascular smooth muscle should be explored. For this purpose, it would be essential to use some vessels that did, and others that did not, have functioning nerve terminals. It would be important here to include studies on selected coronary vessels and on vessels which play a dominant role in the regulation of systemic vascular resistance.

· A number of related studies are needed before the effects on humans can be explained in full, particularly the effects of Δ-9-THC on the renin-angiotensin system in the kidney, which provides control of arterial pressure, and on the several sequences of prostaglandin metabolism.

Studies also are indicated to obtain new data about the effects of marijuana on:

· persons with hypertension, coronary artery disease, and cerebrovascular disease;

· increases in systemic arterial pressure in low- and high-renin hypertension and the interactions between Δ-9-THC and several classes of antihypertensive medications;

· the interactions between the salt and water-retaining effect of Δ-9-THC and diuretics that could be employed both in hypertensives and those with heart failure.

Additionally, studies should be done on the use of standard monitoring techniques to quantify any effect of marijuana smoking on tendencies toward arrhythmias, and on interactions of Δ-9-THC with drugs that modify synaptic transmission in the central nervous system.

REFERENCES

Adams, M.D., Earnhardt, J.T., Dewey, W.L., and Harris, L.S. Vasoconstrictor actions of Δ-8- and Δ-9-tetrahydrocannabinol in the rat. J. Pharmacol. Exp. Ther. 196:649-656, 1976.

Ames, F. A clinical and metabolic study of acute intoxication with cannabis sativa and its role in the model psychoses. J. Ment. Sci. 104:972-999, 1968.

Aronow, W.S. and Cassidy, J. Effect of marihuana and placebo-marihuana smoking on angina pectoris. N. Engl. J. Med. 291:65-67, 1974.

Auerbach, O., Stout, A.P., Hammond, E.C., and Garfinkel, L. Changes in bronchial epithelium relation to cigarette smoking and in relation to lung cancer. N. Engl. J. Med. 265:253-267, 1961.

Beaconsfield, P., Ginsburg, J., and Rainsbury, R. Marihuana smoking: Cardiovascular effects in man and possible mechanisms. N. Engl. J. Med. 287:209-212, 1972.

Bellville, J.W., Swanson, G.D., and Aqleh, K.A. Respiratory effects of Δ-9-tetrahydrocannabinol. Clin. Pharmacol. Ther. 17:541-548, 1975.

Benowitz, N.L. and Jones, R.T. Cardiovascular effects of prolonged Δ-9-tetrahydrocannabinol ingestion. Clin. Pharmacol. Ther. 18:287-297, 1975.

Benowitz, N.L. and Jones, R.T. Effects of Δ-9-tetrahydrocannabinol on drug distribution and metabolism. Clin. Pharmacol. Ther. 22:259-268, 1977a.

Benowitz, N.L. and Jones, R.T. Prolonged Δ-9-tetrahydrocannabinol ingestion: Effects of sympathomimetic amines and autonomic blockades. Clin. Pharmacol. Ther. 21:336-342, 1977b.

Benowitz, N.L., Rosenberg, J., Rogers, W., et al. Cardiovascular effects of intravenous Δ-9-tetrahydrocannabinol: Autonomic nervous mechanisms. Clin. Pharmacol. Ther. 25:440-446, 1979.

Bernstein, J.G., Becker, D., Babor, T.F., and Mendelson, J.H. Physiological assessments: Cardiopulmonary function, pp. 147-160. In Mendelson, J.H., Rossi, A.M., and Meyers, R.E. (eds.) The Use of Marijuana: A Psychological and Physiological Inquiry. New York: Plenum Press, 1974.

Birmingham, M.K. and Bartova, A. Effects of cannabinol derivatives on blood pressure, body weight, pituitary-adrenal function, and mitochondrial respiration in the rat, pp. 425-438. In Nahas, G.G. (ed.) Marihuana: Chemistry, Biochemistry, and Cellular Effects. New York: Springer-Verlag, 1976.

Boulougouris, J.C., Panayiotopoulos, C.P., Antypas, E., et al. Effect of chronic hashish use on medical status in 44 users compared with 38 controls. Ann. N.Y. Acad. Sci. 282:168-172, 1976.

Bright, T.P., Kiplinger, G.F., Brown, D., et al. Effects of beta-adrenergic blockade on marihuana-induced tachycardia, pp. 1737-1744. In Report of the 33rd Annual Scientific Meeting of the Committee on Problems of Drug Dependence. Vol. 2. Washington, D.C.: National Academy of Sciences, 1971.

Burstein, S. and Raz, A. Inhibition of prostaglandin E_2 biosynthesis by Δ-1-tetrahydrocannabinol. Prostaglandins 2:369-374, 1972.

Busch, F.W., Seid, D.A., and Wei, E.T. Mutagenic activity of marihuana smoke condensates. Cancer Lett. 6:319-324, 1979.

Cavero, I., Buckley, J.P., and Jandhyala, B.S. Parasympatholytic activity of (-)-delta-9-transtetrahydrocannabinol in mongrel dogs. Eur. J. Pharmacol. 19:301-304, 1972.

Cavero, I., Solomon, T., Buckley, J.P., and Jandhyala, B.S. Studies on the bradycardia induced by (-)-Δ-9-transtetrahydrocannabinol in anesthetized dogs. Eur. J. Pharmacol. 22:263-269, 1973.

Dornbush, R.L. and Kokkevi, A. Acute effects of cannabis on cognitive, perceptual, and motor performance in chronic hashish users. Ann. N.Y. Acad. Sci. 282:313-322, 1976.

Drath, D.B., Shorey, J.M., Price, L., and Huber, G.L. Metabolic and functional characteristics of alveolar macrophages recovered from rats exposed to marijuana smoke. Infec. Immun. 25:268-272, 1979.

Englert, L.F., Ho, B.T., and Taylor, D. The effects of (-)-Δ-9-tetrahydrocannabinol on reserpine induced hypothermia in rats. Br. J. Pharmacol. 49:243-252, 1973.

Fleischman, R.W., Baker, J.R., and Rosenkrantz, H. Pulmonary pathologic changes in rats exposed to marihuana smoke for 1 year. Toxicol. Appl. Pharmacol. 47:557-566, 1979.

Gash, A., Karliner, J.S., Janowsky, D., and Lake, C.R. Effects of smoking marihuana on left ventricular performance and plasma norepinephrine: Studies in normal men. Ann. Intern. Med. 89:448-452, 1978.

Gill, E.W. and Paton, W.D.M. Pharmacological experiments in vitro on the active principles of cannabis, pp. 165-173. In Joyce, C.R.B., Curry, S.H., London, J., and Churchill, A. The Botany and Chemistry of Cannabis, 1970.

Glatt, H., Ohlsson, A., Agurell, S., and Oesch, F. Δ-1-tetrahydrocannabinol and 1-alpha, 2-alpha-epoxyhexahydrocannabinol: Mutagenicity investigation in the Ames test. Mutat. Res. 66:329-335, 1979.

Graham, J.D.P. and Li, D.M.F. Cardiovascular and respiratory effects of cannabis in cat and rat. Br. J. Pharmacol. 49:1-10, 1973.

Hall, J.A.S. Testimony in Marihuana-Hashish Epidemic Hearing of the Committee of the Judiciary U.S. Senate. Washington, D.C.: U.S. Government Printing Office, 1975.

Hardman, H.F. and Hosko, M.J. An overview of the cardiovascular-autonomic action of cannabis, pp. 231-238. In Braude, M.C. and Szara, S. (eds.) Pharmacology of Marihuana. New York: Raven Press, 1976.

Henderson, R.L., Tennant, F.S., and Guerry, R. Respiratory manifestations of hashish smoking. Arch. Otolaryngol. 95:248-251, 1972.

Hernandez-Bolanos, J., Swenson, E.W., and Coggins, W.J. Preservation of pulmonary function in regular, heavy, long-term marijuana smokers. Am. Rev. Resp. Dis. 113 (Suppl.):100, 1976.

Ho, B.T., Taylor, D., and Englert, L.F. The effect of repeated administration of (-)-Δ-9-tetrahydrocannabinol on the biosynthesis of brain amines. Res. Commun. Chem. Pathol. Pharmacol. 5:851-854, 1973.

Ho, B.T. and Johnson, K.M. Sites of neurochemical action of Δ-9-tetrahydrocannabinol: Interaction with reserpine, pp. 367-382. In Nahas, G.G. (ed.) Marihuana: Chemistry, Biochemistry, and Cellular Effects. New York: Springer-Verlag, 1976.

Hoffmann, D., Brunnemann, K.D., Gori, G.B., and Wynder, E.L. On the carcinogenicity of marijuana smoke, pp. 63-81. In Runeckles, V.C. (ed.) Recent Advances in Phytochemistry New York: Plenum Publishing Corporation, 1975.

Howes, J. and Osgood, P. The effect of Δ-9-tetrahydrocannabinol on the uptake and release of ^{14}C-dopamine from crude striatal synaptosomal preparations. Neuropharmacology 13:1109-1114, 1974.

Howes, J.F. and Osgood, P.F. Cannabinoids and the inhibition of prostaglandin synthesis, pp. 415-424. In Nahas, G.G. (ed.) Marihuana: Chemistry, Biochemistry, and Cellular Effects. New York: Springer-Verlag, 1976.

Huber, G.L., Simmons, G.A., McCarthy, C.R., et al. Depressant effect of marihuana smoke on antibactericidal activity of pulmonary alveolar macrophages. Chest 68:769-773, 1975.

Huber, G.L., Pochay, V.E., Shea, J.W., et al. An experimental animal model for quantifying the biologic effects of marijuana on the defense system of the lung, pp. 301-328. In Nahas, G.G. and Paton, W.D.M. (eds.) Marihuana: Biological Effects. Analysis, Metabolism, Cellular Responses, Reproduction and Brain. Oxford: Pergamon Press, 1979a.

Huber, G.L., Shea, J.W., Hinds, W.E., et al. The gas phase of marijuana smoke and intrapulmonary bactericidal defenses. Bull. Eur. Physiopath. Resp. 15:491-503, 1979b.

Huber, G.L., Pochay, V.E., Pereira, W., et al. Marijuana, tetrahydrocannabinol, and pulmonary antibacterial defenses. Chest 77:403-410, 1980.

Huot, J. Cellular and biochemical alterations induced in vitro by delta-1-tetrahydrocannabinol: Effects on cell proliferation, nucleic acids, plasma cell membrane ATPase, and adenylate cyclase, pp. 313-327. In Nahas, G.G. (ed.) Marihuana: Chemistry, Biochemistry, and Cellular Effects. New York: Springer-Verlag, 1976.

Joachimoglu, G. Natural and smoked hashish, pp. 2-14. In Wolstenholme, G.E.W., Knight, J., London, J., and Churchill, A. Hashish: Its Chemistry and Pharmacology (CIBA Foundation Study Group 21), 1965.

Johnson, S. and Domino, E.F. Some cardiovascular effects of marihuana smoking in normal volunteers. Clin. Pharmacol. Ther. 12:762-768, 1971.

Kanakis, C.J., Pouget, J.M., and Rosen, K.M. The effects of Δ-9-tetrahydrocannabinol (cannabis) on cardiac performance with and without beta blockage. Circulation 53:703-707, 1976.

Kawasaki, H., Watanabe, S., Oishi, R., and Ueki, S. Effects of Δ-9-tetrahydrocannabinol on the cardiovascular system, and pressor and behavioral responses to brain stimulation in rats. Jpn. J. Pharmacol. 30:493-502, 1980.

Kochar, M.S. and Hosko, M.J. Electrocardiographic effects of marihuana. JAMA 225:25-27, 1973.

Leuchtenberger, C. and Leuchtenberger, R. Morphological and cytochemical effects of marijuana cigarette smoke on epithelioid cells of lung explants from mice. Nature 234:227-229, 1971.

Leuchtenberger, C., Leuchtenberger, R., and Schneider, A. Effects of marijuana and tobacco smoke on human lung physiology. Nature 241:137-139, 1973a.

Leuchtenberger, C., Leuchtengerger, R., Ritter, U., and Inui, N. Effects of marijuana and tobacco smoke on DNA and chromosomal complement in human lung explants. Nature 242:403-404, 1973b.

Leuchtenberger, C. and Leuchtenberger, R. Cytological and cytochemical studies of the effect of fresh marijuana cigarette smoke on growth and DNA metabolism of animal and human lung cultures, pp. 595-612. In Braude, M.C. and Szara, S. (eds.) Pharmacology of Marihuana. New York: Raven Press, 1976.

Loewe, S. Pharmacological study, pp. 149-220. In The Marihuana Problem in the City of New York: Sociological, Medical, Psychological and Pharmacological Studies. Lancaster, Pa.: Jacques Cattell Press, 1944.

Malit, L.A., Johnstone, R.E., Bourke, D.I., et al. Intravenous Δ-9-tetrahydrocannabinol: Effects on ventilatory control and cardiovascular dynamics. Anesthesiology 42:666-673, 1975.

Martz, R., Brown, D.J., Forney, R.B., et al. Propranolol antagonism of marihuana induced tachycardia. Life Sci. 11:999-1005, 1972.

Merritt, J.C., Crawford, W.J., Alexander, P.C., et al. Effect of marihuana on intraocular and blood pressure in glaucoma. Ophthalmology 87:222-228, 1980.

Nowlan, R. and Cohen, S. Tolerance to marijuana: Heart rate and subjective "high." Clin. Pharmacol. Ther. 22:550-556, 1977.

Perez-Reyes, M., Lipton, M.A., Timmons, M.C., et al. Pharmacology of orally administered Δ-9-tetrahydrocannabinol. Clin. Pharmacol. Ther. 14:48-55, 1973.

Rosenkrantz, H. and Braude, M.C. Acute, subacute and 23-day chronic marihuana inhalation toxicities in the rat. Toxicol. Appl. Pharmacol. 28:428-441, 1974.

Roy, P.E., Magnan-Lapointe, F., Huy, N.D., and Boutet, M. Chronic inhalation of marijuana and tobacco in dogs: Pulmonary pathology. Res. Commun. Chem. Pathol. Pharmacol. 14:305-317, 1976.

Rubin, V. and Comitas, L. Ganja in Jamaica: A Medical Anthropological Study of Chronic Marijuana Use. The Hague: Mouton and Co., 1975.

Seid, D.A. and Wei, E.T. Mutagenic activity of marihuana smoke condensates. Pharmacologist 21:204, 1979.

Shapiro, B.J., Tashkin, D.P., and Frank, I.M. Mechanism of increased specific airway conductance with marijuana smoking in healthy young men. Ann. Int. Med. 78:832-833, 1973.

Shapiro, B.J., Tashkin, D.P., and Frank, I.M. Effects of beta-adrenergic blockade and muscarinic stimulation upon cannabis bronchodilation, pp. 277-286. In Braude, M.C. and Szara, S. (eds.) Pharmacology of Marihuana. New York: Raven Press, 1976a.

Shapiro, B.J., Reiss, S., Sullivan, S.F., Tashkin, D.P., Simmons, M.S., Smith, R.T. Cardiopulmonary effects of marijuana smoking during exercise. Chest 70:441, 1976b.

Stefanis, C. Biological aspects of cannabis use, pp. 149-178. In Petersen, R.C. (ed.) The National Challenge of Drug Abuse. NIDA Research Monograph No. 19. HEW Publication No. (ADM)78-654. Washington, D.C.: U.S. Government Printing Office, 1978.

Sulkowski, A., Vachon, L., and Rich, E.S., Jr. Propranolol effects on acute marihuana intoxication in man. Psychopharmacology 52:47-53, 1977.

Tashkin, D.P., Shapiro, B.J., and Frank, I.M. Acute pulmonary physiologic effects of smoked marijuana and oral Δ-9-tetrahydrocannabinol in healthy young men. N. Engl. J. Med. 289:336-341, 1973.

Tashkin, D.P., Shapiro, B.J., and Frank, I.M. Acute effects of smoked marijuana and oral Δ-9-tetrahydrocannabinol on specific airway conductance in asthmatic subjects. Am. Rev. Respir. Dis. 109:420-428, 1974.

Tashkin, D.P., Shapiro, B.J., Lee, Y.E., and Harper, C.E. Effects of smoked marijuana in experimentally induced asthma. Am. Rev. Respir. Dis. 112:377-386, 1975.

Tashkin, D.P., Shapiro, B.J., Lee, E.Y., Harper, C.E. Subacute effects of heavy marijuana smoking pulmonary function in healthy young males. N. Engl. J. Med. 294:125-129, 1976.

Tashkin, D.P., Reiss, S., Shapiro, B.J., et al. Bronchial effects of aerosolized -9-tetrahydrocannabinol in healthy and asthmatic subjects. Am. Rev. Respir. Dis. 115:57-65, 1977a.

Tashkin, D.P., Levisman, J.A., and Abbasi, A.S. Short-term effects of smoked marihuana on left ventricular function in man. Chest 72:20-26, 1977b.

Tashkin, D.P., Soares, J.R., Hepler, R.S., Shapiro, B.J., and Rachelefsky, G.S. Cannabis, 1977. Ann. Int. Med. 89:539-549, 1978.

Tashkin, D.P., Calvarese, B.M., Simmons, M.S., and Shapiro, B.J. Respiratory status of seventy-four habitual marijuana smokers. Chest 78:699-706, 1980.

Tennant, F.S., Preble, M., Prendergast, T.J., and Ventry, P. Medical manifestations associated with hashish. JAMA 216:1965-1969, 1971.

Tennant, F.S., Guerry, R.L., and Henderson, R.L. Histopathologic and clinical abnormalities of the respiratory system in chronic hashish smokers. Substance and Alcohol Misuse 1:93-100, 1980.

Truitt, E.B. and Anderson, S.M. Biogenic amine alterations produced in the brain by tetrahydrocannabinols and their metabolites. Ann. N.Y. Acad. Sci. 191:68-73, 1971.

Vachon, L., FitzGerald, M.X., Solliday, N.H., et al. Single-dose effect of marihuana smoke: Bronchial dynamics and respiratory-center sensitivity in normal subjects. N. Engl. J. Med. 288:985-989, 1973.

van Went, G.F. Mutagenicity testing of 3 hallucinogens: LSD, psilocybin and Δ-9-THC, using the micronucleus test. Experientia 34:324-325, 1978.

Vollmer, R.R., Cavero, I., Ertel, R.J., et al. Role of the central automatic nervous system in the hypotension and bradycardia induced by (-)-Δ-9-trans-tetrahydrocannabinol. J. Pharm. Pharmacol. 26:186-192, 1974.

Wehner, F.C., Van Rensburg, S.J., and Thiel, P.G. Mutagenicity of marijuana and transkei tobacco smoke condensates in the salmonella/microsome assay. Mutat. Res. 77:135-142, 1980.

Weil, A.T., Zinberg, N.E., and Nelsen, J.M. Clinical and psychological effects of marihuana in man. Science 162:1234-1242, 1968.

Weiss, J.L., Watanabe, A.M., Lemberger, L., et al. Cardiovascular effects of Δ-9-tetrahydrocannabinol in man. Clin. Pharmacol. Ther. 13:671-684, 1972.

Zwillich, C.W., Doekel, R., Hammill, S., and Weil, J.V. The effects of smoked marijuana on metabolism and respiratory control. Am. Rev. Respir. Dis. 118:885-891, 1978.

4

EFFECTS OF MARIJUANA ON THE BRAIN

The most clearly established effects of cannabis are upon behavior.
These effects, described in Chapter 6, indicate that major actions of
cannabinoids are upon the brain. The ways in which marijuana alters
the brain to produce its behavioral effects are not known.

Efforts to discover the causes of the behavioral effects have
included studies on brain morphology, physiology, and chemistry to be
reviewed in this chapter. Effects of marijuana on brain electrical
activity and on brain chemistry have been measured, but their
significance for brain function is not known because of our limited
knowledge of brain-behavior relations. Marijuana causes temporary
intoxication and results in changes in brain physiology and chemistry
similar to those caused by other intoxicating drugs. Although these
kinds of studies may ultimately shed light on the way marijuana
produces its behavioral changes, they do not provide answers to
important clinical questions. Does marijuana cause long-term changes
in the brain that lead to chronic psychiatric or neurological
disorders? So far, the studies reviewed below provide no convincing
evidence for long-term changes because of use of marijuana.

BRAIN MORPHOLOGY

There is substantial controversy about whether marijuana causes
changes in brain structure or in brain cells. Two studies have
reported that marijuana produces changes in brain morphology. Both
suffer sufficiently from methodologic and interpretational defects
that their conclusions cannot be accepted. Furthermore, other
studies have not found changes in morphology.

Gross Morphology

Data suggesting that use of marijuana causes brain atrophy were
obtained by pneumoencephalography (injection of air into spaces in
and surrounding the brain) on 10 users of marijuana who had sought
medical attention because of neurologic complaints (Campbell et al.,
1971). The size of the largest brain cavities (ventricles) was

measured to determine whether loss of brain tissue had occurred. The authors interpreted their data as showing that atrophy was present.

One of the first critics of this report questioned the interpretation of the radiologic techniques used (Bull, 1971). The results also have been seriously criticized because of the marijuana users studied. They had neurological symptoms or signs sufficient to justify an invasive and painful diagnostic test, but there is no evidence that such neurological complaints occur with greater frequency in users of marijuana than in the general population. Further, Campbell's patients did not only use marijuana, but also used such behavior-altering drugs, as lysergic acid diethylamide (LSD) and amphetamines.

More recent evidence has been provided by computed tomography (CT) scans of the brain. This technique, which is noninvasive, painless, and yields more precise and quantifiable measures of brain atrophy, has replaced pneumoencephalography as a diagnostic test. Using CT methods, two studies failed to find evidence of cerebral atrophy in healthy chronic marijuana users (Co et al., 1977; Keuhnle et al., 1977). These latter results suggest that the earlier findings were attributable to the imprecision of conventional pneumoencephalography, or to the fact that a group with neurologic complaints was studied, or to the use of multiple psychoactive drugs by these individuals. This last possibility is reinforced by CT scans of animals who received a variety of psychoactive drugs. Marijuana alone produced no evidence of brain atrophy, whereas other drugs, such as amphetamines, did produce changes (Rumbaugh et al., 1980).

Microscopic Morphology

Three post mortem studies on monkeys in the same laboratory have reported changes in the microscopic morphology of the brain at the ultrastructural level (Harper et al., 1977; Meyers and Heath, 1979; Heath et al., 1980). No similar studies on human beings have been reported. The monkeys received either chronic exposure to marijuana smoke or chronic injections of Δ-9-THC. Changes reported to have occurred in the brains included alteration in synaptic* cleft width, increased density of synaptic cleft material, a decrease in volume of rough endoplasmic reticulum, presence of clumping of synaptic vesicles in axon terminals (where impulses travel away from the cell body), and an increase in intranuclear inclusions. These changes appear dramatic, but they must be interpreted with caution. The three studies are based principally upon examination of two limited brain areas only in three treated monkeys, two receiving marijuana smoke

---

*A synapse is the region of communication between nerve cells, forming the place where a nervous impulse is transmitted from one nerve cell to another.

82

and one intravenous Δ-9-THC; a fourth treated animal was added to
the last study and more brain areas were analyzed in it (Heath et
al., 1980). Further, although the material was evaluated
"doubleblind" after electron micrographs had been made, it would
appear that fixation, tissue preparation, and photography were
carried out before these safeguards against bias were applied. It is
possible that unknown but systematic differences occurred between
experimental (treated) and control animals in fixation and
preparation of tissue or in selection of samples for micrography. In
addition, it should be noted that at least one of the changes noted,
clumping of synaptic vesicles (Harper et al., 1977), is a normal
variant in the synaptic morphology of axon terminals in mammalian
brain (Sipe and Moore, 1977) and does not represent a pathological
change. Also, these studies have not been replicated and, because
the basis for interpretation is such a limited sample, it is concluded that no definitive interpretation can be made at this time.
However, the possibility that marijuana may produce chronic, ultrastructural changes in brain has not been ruled out and should be
investigated.

NEUROPHYSIOLOGY

One source of information on the mechanisms of action of a drug, such
as marijuana, is the study of its physiological effects. Effects of
marijuana on the electrical activity of the brain have been
demonstrated by means of the electroencephalogram (EEG). The
standard, or clinical, EEG measures tiny variations at the scalp of
voltages produced by the electrical activity of the brain. Voltage
differences between two points on the scalp, or between the scalp and
an inactive reference site, are recorded on moving paper, producing a
graph of voltage over time. The waves observed are classified
according to frequencies as delta, theta, alpha, and beta. While the
changes in EEG described below are of interest, their biological
significance is unknown.

Acute (Short-Term) Effects in Waking EEG

Ingested marijuana or Δ-9-THC produces rather slight effects on the
EEG of an awake subject. Relatively high doses (210 mg Δ-9-THC or
its equivalent/day) have failed to produce measurable changes even
though marked behavioral effects were observed. The EEG effect most
frequently reported in recent studies has been an increased abundance
of alpha waves associated with a slight slowing (about 0.25 Hz) of
the alpha frequency (Rodin et al., 1970; Volavka et al., 1971; Fink,
1976). However, reduced alpha abundance and increased fast frequency
activity (beta) have also been reported (Wikler and Lloyd, 1945;
Jones and Stone, 1970). Most studies which report EEG changes have
noted that tolerance develops with repeated drug administration. No
significance with respect to hazard can be inferred from the effects

of cannabis on the waking EEG. For a further review of this
literature, see Fried (1977).

Persistent Effects in Waking EEG

The occurrence of persistent (long-lasting) changes in EEG with use
of marijuana would cause concern even if their significance for brain
function was unknown. However, in attempting to investigate the
question of whether such changes occur, there inevitably arise crucial
issues of subject selection. If one selects only chronic marijuana
users who are in good health, one may be eliminating systematically
those who have been adversely affected by use of the drug and who
might have shown EEG changes. On the other hand, if one includes in
such studies marijuana users who suffer from various illnesses or
behavioral disturbances, one might find abnormalities of the EEG that
result from these conditions rather than from the marijuana.

Long-term use of marijuana, either in the modest doses customarily used in this country or the heavy doses of hashish and ganga
used by certain studied populations abroad, has not been shown to
produce changes in the EEG. No abnormalities were found in the EEG
of 10 healthy students who had smoked marijuana regularly for 1 year
(Rodin et al., 1970). Another study compared clinical EEG records of
46 hashish users and 40 matched controls in Greece (Fink, 1976).
Each record was evaluated independently by four qualified neurologist-
electroencephalographers. No differences were observed in the
incidence of abnormal records in the users and controls, a result
consistent with the absence of significant differences between the
two groups in various tests of neurological function.

Essentially, the same negative results were obtained in studies
of ganga users in Jamaica (Rubin and Comitas, 1975) and marijuana
users in Costa Rica (Karacan et al., 1976). In these later studies
subjects were carefully selected to include only those in good health
who were functioning adequately in the community. As mentioned above,
this method of selection runs the risk of eliminating subjects whose
health or behavior were adversely affected by marijuana and who might
have shown EEG changes. This methodological difficulty cannot be
eliminated in any small sample investigation of marijuana users.

Acute Effects in Event-Related Potentials

One can employ computer averaging to retrieve from the EEG certain
information that is not detectable by visual inspection. In this
way, the electrical events that follow a stimulus may be studied in
subjects who are at rest, asleep, or carrying out certain tasks.
These computer-averaged potentials provide clues to the sequential
processing of information by the brain.

Although the literature is inconsistent, it is clear that cannabis
can produce effects on event-related potentials (EPs) (Herning et
al., 1979). Effects on amplitude are more often reported than effects

on latency of the event-related waves. Several studies with inconsistent results have appeared; these inconsistencies result from differences in task, dose, or duration of administration. Thus, EPs in response to sensory stimuli are unaffected or even increased by cannabis if the subject is passive, but are decreased in amplitude if the subject is performing a task. One study found the first negative wave, a component of the auditory EP, was reduced at a dose of 180-210 mg per day, but not at a dose of 70-90 mg per day during acute (1 to 3 days) administration (Herning et al., 1979). After 2 weeks at the higher dosage, this effect was observed only for the more difficult tasks. This study demonstrates differences in marijuana effects on EPs according to dose, duration of administration, and task complexity.

Acute Effects in Sleep EEG

Drugs often produce marked effects on the EEG during sleep, but producing little or no change in the waking EEG. This is the case with marijuana and Δ-9-THC.

In relatively high doses (70-210 mg/day), Δ-9-THC and marijuana extract produced marked effects on sleep EEG (Feinberg et al., 1975, 1976). On initial administration, the time spent in REM sleep* (stage REM duration) was reduced below baseline levels (placebo) by 18 percent and the number of eye movements by 49 percent. Some tolerance (return toward baseline levels) was apparent during the period (12-16 days) of drug administration. On withdrawal, REM duration was increased above baseline by 49 percent and rapid eye movements were increased by 67 percent. While these effects are quite large, their clinical significance is unknown. They were not accompanied by such unusual behavioral changes as hallucinations or disorientation, although there was evidence of withdrawal—irritability, increased reflexes, and mild agitation. With much smaller doses of Δ-9-THC, either a small reduction in REM sleep (Pivik et al., 1972; Freemon, 1974) or no change has been reported (Barratt et al., 1974; Hosko et al., 1973; Pranikoff et al., 1973).

Persistent Effects in Sleep EEG

We are not aware of any investigation of sleep in abstinent long-term marijuana users. However, 32 male chronic marijuana users and matched controls were studied in Costa Rica (Karacan et al., 1976). The users habitually smoked 2.5 to 23.3 cigarettes per day (mean = 9.2) and had used the drug for 10 to 27 years; they continued their usual intake during the study (Costa Rican cigarettes contain about 200 mg

---

*A stage in sleep during which Rapid Eye Movements may be detected and vivid dreaming usually occurs.

of marijuana). The subjects selected for this study had normal medical, neurologic, and laboratory evaluations.

Sleep was recorded for 8 consecutive nights. Prior to each night's recording, the users described their marijuana intake during the previous 24 hours. This intake was not directly monitored or controlled by the experimenters, because the goal was to observe sleep patterns under "naturalistic" conditions. The subjects were forbidden to use marijuana during the 2-3 hours prior to sleep recording. (For further details of this extensive study, see Karacan et al., 1976.)

All of the major variables derived from visual sleep stage classification were examined. The only statistically significant differences between marijuana users and their matched controls were in one of the sleep latency measures and in REM percentage of total sleep and average REM period length. The differences were quite small and may have been due to the subjects experiencing early withdrawal at the time their sleep was recorded. This is a likely explanation for these findings according to studies described previously (Feinberg et al., 1975, 1976).

The Costa Rican study concluded there was a lack of evidence of major disturbances of EEG sleep patterns in user subjects studied in situ (Karacan et al., 1976). Thus, long-term marijuana use has not been demonstrated to cause marked and consistent abnormalities of sleep EEG that can be demonstrated in studies with small samples.

Electrophysiological Studies in Animals

Sleep Studies

The findings of several animal studies carried out to investigate the effects of marijuana on EEG differ in some respects to those in human beings. Species differences are thought to be responsible for some of the variations found from species to species. For example, 5 and 10 mg/kg Δ-9-THC administered acutely to rats suppressed REM, reduced slow-wave sleep, and increased wakefulness (Moreton and Davis, 1973). Chronic administration caused an initial suppression of REM, which returned to baseline after 4 days and remained at baseline levels for a further 16 days. In contrast to the human studies, there was no withdrawal increase in REM above baseline during a 10-day withdrawal period. Similar results were obtained in a short-term study that employed intravenous doses of Δ-9-THC (0.5 and 1.0 mg/kg) to rabbits (Fujuimori and Himwich, 1973).

Appreciable qualitative differences in sleep EEG response to Δ-9-THC have also been detected in primates when compared with human studies. When 1.2 mg/kg Δ-9-THC is administered to squirrel monkeys in a single oral dose, daily for 60 days, no significant effects on REM sleep duration occurred; instead, a decrease in EEG stages 3 and 4 was noted (Adams and Barratt, 1975).

EEG Studies in Subcortical Structures

Electrode implantation is rarely possible in man, but is a routine and essential technique for the study of brain electrophysiology in animals. Animal experiments also permit use of higher doses and more prolonged administration than is possible with human subjects. For these reasons, animal experiments can yield important data that cannot be obtained in human studies. In general, EEG recordings after short-term administration of marijuana are similar from surface (cortex) or from deep brain (subcortex) regions. However, after chronic administration of high doses of Δ-9-THC, abnormal recordings have been observed in subcortical regions of some animals, readings not seen in the cortex. Although these findings have not been replicated, they are of particular concern, because they raise the possibility that chronic exposure to high doses of marijuana produces long-lasting effects on brain physiology.

After intravenous administration of a range of Δ-9-THC doses (from 0.05 to 12.8 mg/kg) to rhesus monkeys, a general increase in EEG synchrony was observed; and at higher dose ranges, there were specific EEG changes in the limbic system, frontal cortex, thalamus and fastigial nuclei (Martinez et al., 1972). In this study, the increase in high-voltage activity showed a good dose-response relationship. In a second study, oral dosing of three rhesus monkeys with a crude marijuana extract containing 25 percent Δ-9-THC produced dose-related EEG changes, including slow waves in the hippocampus, amygdala, and septum (Stadnicki et al., 1974). Tolerance to the behavioral and EEG changes occurred with daily treatment, which was stopped after 51 days. Behavioral withdrawal effects were noted, but EEG changes during withdrawal were minimal and there was no evidence of EEG changes persisting beyond the period of Δ-9-THC ingestion.

Two studies that monitored EEG recording from deep brain sites after chronic administration of high doses of marijuana found changes in EEGs from deep brain sites that were not observed in surface areas after drug withdrawal (Fehr et al., 1976; Heath, 1976; Heath et al., 1979). Studies of two rats with electrodes implanted in the anterior neocortex, dorsal hippocampus, and mesencephalic reticular formation 1 year after exposure to 20 mg/kg for 6 months (Fehr et al., 1976) yielded hippocampal recordings with "epileptiform" abnormalities, in contrast to one control and two alcohol-treated animals.

The second study was carried out on thirteen feral-raised rhesus monkeys (Heath 1976; Heath et al., 1979). Ten monkeys had electrodes implanted in deep sites and in brain cortex. Four monkeys were made to smoke marijuana three times a day, 5 days per week for 6 months; two other monkeys with implants were given 0.6 mg/kg Δ-9-THC each day, 5 days per week for 6 months; still other monkeys were used as controls or received smaller doses of marijuana. In three high-dose monkeys, two smoking and one ingesting Δ-9-THC, changes in EEG could be detected in recordings from deep brain sites; the changes continued 7 months after cessation of marijuana exposure. No EEG abnormalities were present in recordings from the brain surface.

One of the major criticisms of both these studies is their use of small numbers of animals. Furthermore, there have been no attempts at replication by other workers. Nevertheless, because these findings provide some of the only evidence for a possible irreversible effect of chronic high doses of marijuana, they are mentioned here with a strong urging for additional studies in an effort to replicate these findings.

EPILEPSY

Because of the effects of marijuana on brain electrical activity, questions have been raised about its association with epilepsy. Two questions are raised in the literature. First, does marijuana produce seizures? Second, does marijuana or a derivative prevent seizures? The first question will be discussed here. The second is reviewed in Chapter 7, which is concerned with the potential therapeutic uses of cannabis.

There are anecdotal reports in the literature that suggest seizures may be induced by marijuana in some persons with a known seizure disorder. A rigorous study, using adequate numbers of patients with documented seizure patterns, has not been done. Reports of experimental animal studies are conflicting and varied (Feeney et al., 1973, 1979; Lemberger, 1980). There are some circumstances in which cannabis administration does not alter certain types of seizures such as the photosensitive seizures in the baboon (Meldrum et al., 1974), and others in which it seems that seizures are induced. A single rabbit that responded to Δ-9-THC adminis- tration with seizures was bred to establish a colony of rabbits with similar response (Consroe and Fish, 1981). It will be of consider- able interest to determine mechanisms of seizure induction and pharmacologic response patterns in this unusual animal model. However, as described further in Chapter 7, the bulk of the animal literature and some data from human studies suggest that the more prominent effect of marijuana derivatives, especially cannabinol and cannabidiol, is to decrease rather than increase seizure suscepti- bility (see Karler and Turkanis, 1981, for review).

NEUROCHEMISTRY

Our knowledge of the effects of marijuana on brain chemistry has come largely from studies in animals. Cannabis and some of its derivatives have been shown to cause chemical effects in the brain, as demonstrated by effects on neurotransmitters and on nucleic acids. The evidence is reviewed below.

Neurotransmitters

The brain is composed of many information-processing networks of nerve cells. Within each of these networks the transfer of information from one nerve cell to another is dependent upon chemicals called neurotransmitters. These substances are produced by nerve cells, released when the cells are stimulated and act to alter the excitability of neighboring nerve cells. Neurotransmitters play an essential role in the transmission and processing of information, and it is not surprising that many drugs that alter behavior do so by their actions on neurotransmitters. The understanding of the effects of marijuana on the brain must include knowledge of its effects on neurotransmitter systems.

Several different classes of chemicals act as neurotransmitters. The first chemical to be demonstrated to have this function was acetylcholine, and it is now established that acetylcholine is the neurotransmitter for several nerve cell networks in the brain. A number of studies in animals have examined the effect of marijuana on brain acetylcholine (see Domino, 1981, for a brief review of the extensive literature). The most clear-cut effects have been on acetylcholine turnover, a measure of the level of activity of neurons producing the chemical. Small doses of Δ-9-THC cause a reduction in acetylcholine turnover in the hippocampus (Domino et al., 1978; Revuelta et al., 1978; Domino, 1981) and this results from reduced activity of the acetylcholine neurons. It is noteworthy that the effect is produced by small doses and only by cannabinoids. Administration of physostigmine, a drug that enhances acetylcholine action by partially blocking its breakdown, to five healthy human volunteers (2 hours after ingestion of 20 to 40 mg of Δ-9-THC) produced enhancement of the lethargy and somnolence occurring late in the course of the Δ-9-THC intoxication (Freemon et al., 1975). The results of this study, and others in man and animals (El-Yousef et al., 1973; Low et al., 1973; Drew and Miller, 1974; Freemon et al., 1975), have led to the conclusion that Δ-9-THC acts to inhibit acetylcholine nerve cell networks. The exact nature of this action is not known, but it may be related to the memory deficits produced (Domino, 1981).

There have been studies of cannabinoids on several other neurotransmitters in brain, including catecholamines, serotonin, and gamma aminobutyric acid (Banerjee et al., 1975; Bracs et al., 1975). Although some effects have been reported, they either are produced by a very high dose or are so fragmentary that their implications are unclear. The effects of cannabinoids on neurotransmitters that have been studied to date, other than acetylcholine, are not striking. In particular, there is no evidence for any significant, long-term toxic effect of cannabinoids on any of the nerve cell networks that produce identified neurotransmitters.

Proteins, Enzymes, Nucleic Acids

A very few studies have examined the effects of marijuana on neurochemical variabless other than neurotransmitters (Luthra and Rosenkrantz, 1974; Luthra et al., 1975, 1976). After chronic administration to rats either of Δ-9-THC or marijuana smoke (for

periods from 28 to 180 days), these investigators examined brain
lipid, protein, and ribonucleic acid (RNA) content. With very high
doses of Δ-9-THC (up to 500 mg/kg/day), some decrease in brain
protein and RNA was noted; no decrease was noted in lipid content.
However, with smaller doses, or administration of marijuana smoke, no
consistent or marked changes were noted. The significance of these
effects is unknown. Whether additional effects might be observed
with more sophisticated and sensitive methods directed to more
restricted analytical problems cannot be answered at present.

SUMMARY

There is no persuasive evidence that marijuana causes morphological
changes in the brain. Computer tomography studies on users of
marijuana reveal no gross changes in brain structure. Electron
micrographic studies of monkey brains indicating morphologic changes
are methodologically flawed and cannot be used as evidence for an
effect of marijuana on brain cell morphology. Clear effects on brain
electrical activity in human beings and in animals have been found
after drug exposure. These effects have not been demonstrated to
persist in human beings after the drug has been discontinued.
Studies of EEG from deep brain structures in chronically treated
animals have shown changes after the withdrawl of the drug. These
limited findings need to be confirmed by further studies. Studies in
human beings and animals indicate that, despite the neurophysiologic
effects demonstrated in EEG studies, marijuana does not appear to
increase epileptic seizure susceptibility. Current evidence has
shown marijuana causes some chemical changes in brain. Cannabinoids
affect several neurotransmitter systems, especially the cholinergic
system. At high doses marijuana also has been shown to affect
nucleoprotein synthesis. The significance of these findings for
brain function as demonstrated by human behavior or their clinical
relevance is unknown.

RECOMMENDATIONS FOR RESEARCH

In view of the widespread use of cannabis, it would be worthwhile to
carry out further and more systematic studies of the effects of
cannabis on brain structure, chemistry, and electrophysiology. Such
studies should be closely correlated with behavior, e.g., learning,
psychomotor coordination (see Chapter 6). One useful approach might
be to investigate the effects of medium and high doses of cannabis
(defined in terms of the patterns of human consumption) on juvenile
and adult monkeys during and after long-term exposure. Juvenile
monkeys should be included because the immature nervous system may be
more sensitive to harmful drug effects; this issue is of great
clinical concern, because marijuana use by human beings now begins
quite early in life (see Chapter 2). Observations also should be
made during long-term abstinence after previous long-term exposure to

determine whether any persistent abnormalities have been produced. A systematic approach to these questions using modern methods of measurement and analysis could extend our present knowledge substantially.

REFERENCES

Adams, P.M. and Barratt, E.S. Effect of chronic marijuana administration on stages of primate sleepwakefulness. Biol. Psychiatry 10:315-322, 1975.

Banerjee, S.P., Snyder, S.H., and Mechoulam, R. Cannabinoids: Influence on neurotransmitter uptake in rat brain synaptosomes. J. Pharmacol. Exp. Ther. 194:74-81, 1975.

Barratt, E.S., Beaver, W., and White, R. The effects of marijuana on human sleep patterns. Biol. Psychiatry 8:47-54, 1974.

Bracs, P., Jackson, D.M., and Chester, G.B. The effect of Δ-9-tetrahydrocannabinol on brain amine concentration and turnover in whole rat brain and in various regions of the brain. J. Pharm. Pharmacol. 27:713-715, 1975.

Bull, J. Cerebral atrophy in young cannabis smokers. Lancet 2:1420, 1971.

Campbell, A.M.G., Evans, M., Thomson, J.L.G., and Williams, M.J. Cerebral atrophy in young cannabis smokers. Lancet 2:1219-1225, 1971.

Co, B.T., Goodwin, D.N., Gado, M., et al. Absence of cerebral atrophy in chronic cannabis users. JAMA 237:1229-1230, 1977.

Consroe, P. and Fish, B.S. Behavioral pharmacology of tetrahydrocannabinol convulsions in rabbits. Comm. Psychopharmacol. Comm. Pharmacol. 4:287-291, 1981.

Domino, E.F., Donelson, A.C., and Tuttle, T. Effects of Δ-9-tetrahydrocannabinol on regional brain acetylcholine, pp. 673-678. In Jenden, D.J. (ed.) Cholinergic Mechanisms and Psychopharmacology. New York: Plenum Press, 1978.

Domino, E.F. Cannabinoids and the cholinergic system. J. Clin. Pharmacol. 21(Suppl.):249S-255S, 1981.

Drew, W.G. and Miller, L.L. Cannabis: Neural mechanisms and behavior--A theoretical review. Pharmacology 11:12-32, 1974.

El-Yousef, M.K., Janowsky, D.S., Davis, J.M., and Rosenblatt, J.E. Induction of severe depression by physostigmine in marijuana intoxicated individuals. Br. J. Addict. 68:321-325, 1973.

Fehr, K.A., Kalant, H., Leblanc, A.E., and Knox, G.V. Permanent learning impairment after chronic heavy exposure to cannabis or ethanol in the rat, pp. 495-505. In Nahas, G.G. (ed.) Marihuana: Chemistry, Biochemistry, and Cellular Effects. New York: Springer-Verlag, 1976.

Feeney, D.M., Wagner, H.R., McNamara, M.C., and Weiss, G. Effects of tetrahydrocannabinol on hippocampal evoked afterdischarges in cats. Exp. Neurol. 41:357-365, 1973.

Feeney, D.M. Marihuana and epilepsy: Paradoxical anticonvulsant and convulsant effects, pp. 643-657. In Nahas, G.G. and Paton,

W.D.M. (eds.) Marihuana: Biological Effects. Analysis, Metabolism, Cellular Responses, Reproduction and Brain. Oxford: Pergamon Press, 1979.

Feinberg, I., Jones, R., Walker, J.M., et al. Effects of high dosage delta-9-tetrahydrocannabinol on sleep patterns in man. Clin. Pharmacol. Ther. 17:458-466, 1975.

Feinberg, I., Jones, R., Walker, J.M., et al. Effects of marijuana tetrahydrocannabinol on electroencephalographic sleep patterns. Clin. Pharmacol. Ther. 19:782-794, 1976.

Fink, M. Effects of acute and chronic inhalation of hashish, marijuana, and delta-9-tetrahydrocannabinol on brain electrical activity in man: Evidence for tissue tolerance. Ann. N.Y. Acad. Sci. 282:387-398, 1976.

Freemon, F.R. The effect of delta-9-tetrahydrocannabinol on sleep. Psychopharmacologia 35:39-44, 1974.

Freemon, F.R., Rosenblatt, J.E., and El-Yousef, M.K. Interaction of physostigmine and delta-9-tetrahydrocannabinol in man. Clin. Pharmacol. Ther. 17:121-126, 1975.

Fried, P.A. Behavioral and electroencephalographic correlates of the chronic use of marijuana--A review. Behav. Biol. 21:163-196, 1977.

Fujimori, M. and Himwich, H.E. Δ-9-Tetrahydrocannabinol and the sleep-wakefulness cycle in rabbits. Physiol. Behav. 11:291-295, 1973.

Harper, J.W., Heath, R.G., and Myers, W.A. Effects of cannabis sativa on ultrastructure of the synapse in monkey brain. J. Neurosci. Res. 3:87-93, 1977.

Heath, R.G. Marihuana and Δ-9-tetrahydrocannabinol: Acute and chronic effects on brain function of monkeys, pp. 345-356. In Braude, M.C. and Szara, S. (eds.) Pharmacology of Marihuana. New York: Raven Press, 1976.

Heath, R.G., Fitzjarrell, A.T., Garey, R.E., and Myers, W.A. Chronic marihuana smoking: Its effect on function and structure of the primate brain, pp. 713-730. In Nahas, G.G. and Paton, W.D.M. (eds.) Marihuana: Biological Effects. Analysis, Metabolism, Cellular Responses, Reproduction and Brain. Oxford: Pergamon Press, 1979.

Heath, R.G., Fitzjarrell, A.T., Fontana, C.J., and Garey, R.E. Cannabis sativa: Effects on brain function and ultrastructure in Rhesus monkeys. Biol. Psychiatry 15:657-690, 1980.

Herning, R.I., Jones, R.T., and Peltzman, D.J. Changes in human event related potentials with prolonged delta-9-tetrahydrocannabinol (THC) use. Electroencephalogr. Clin. Neurophysiol. 47:556-570, 1979.

Hosko, M.J., Kochar, M.S., and Wang, R.I.H. Effects of orally administered delta-9-tetrahydrocannabiol in man. Clin. Pharmacol. Ther. 14:344-352, 1973.

Jones, R.T. and Stone, G.C. Psychological studies of marijuana and alcohol in man. Psychopharmacologia 18:108-117, 1970.

Karacan, I., Fernandez-Salas, A., Coggins, W.J., et al. Sleep electroencephalographic-electrooculographic characteristics of chronic marijuana users: Part I. Ann. N.Y. Acad. Sci. 282:348-374, 1976.

Karler, R. and Turkanis, S.A. The cannabinoids as potential antiepileptics. J. Clin. Pharmacol. 21(Suppl.):4375-4485, 1981.

Kuehnle, J., Mendelson, J.H., Davis, K.R., and New, P.F.J. Computed tomographic examination of heavy marijuana smokers. JAMA 237:1231-1232, 1977.

Lemberger, L. Potential therapeutic usefulness of marijuana. Ann. Rev. Pharmacol. Toxicol. 20:151-172, 1980.

Low, M.D., Klonoff, H., and Marcus, A. The neurophysiological basis of the marijuana experience. Can. Med. Assoc. J. 108:157-164, 1973.

Luthra, Y.K. and Rosenkrantz, H. Cannabinoids: Neurochemical aspects after oral chronic administration to rats. Toxicol. Appl. Pharmacol. 27:158-168, 1974.

Luthra, Y.K., Rosenkrantz, H., Heyman, I.A., and Braude, M.C. Differential neurochemistry and temporal pattern in rats treated orally with Δ-9-tetrahydrocannabinol for periods up to six months. Toxicol. Appl. Pharmacol. 32:418-431, 1975.

Luthra, Y.K., Rosenkrantz, H., and Braude, M.C. Cerebral and cerebellar neurochemical changes and behavioral manifestations in rats chronically exposed to marijuana smoke. Toxicol. Appl. Pharmacol. 35:455-465, 1976.

Martinez, J.L., Stadnicki, S.W., and Schaeppi, U.N. Delta-9-tetrahydrocannabinol: Effects on EEG and behavior of Rhesus monkeys. Life Sci. 11:643-651, 1972.

Meldrum, B.S., Fariello, R.G., Puil, E.A., et al. Delta-9-tetrahydrocannabinol and epilepsy in the photosensitive baboon, Papio papio. Epilepsia 15:255-264, 1974.

Moreton, J.E. and Davis, W.M. Electroencephalographic study of the effects of tetrahydrocannabinols on sleep in the rat. Neuropharmacology 12:897-907, 1973.

Myers, W.A. and Heath, R.G. Cannabis sativa: Ultrastructural changes in organelles of neurons in brain septal region of monkeys. J. Neurosci. Res. 4:9-17, 1979.

Pivik, R.T., Zarcone, V., Dement, W.C., and Hollister, L.E. Delta-9-tetrahydrocannabinol and synhexl: Effects on human sleep patterns. Clin. Pharmacol. Ther. 13:426-435, 1972.

Pranikoff, K., Karacan, I., Larson, E.A., et al. Effects of marijuana smoking on the sleep EEG: Preliminary studies. J. Fla. Med. Assoc. 60:28-31, 1973.

Revuelta, A.V., Moroni, F., Cheney, D.L., and Costa, E. Effect of cannabinoids on the turnover rate of acetylcholine in rat hippocampus, striatum, and cortex. Arch. Pharmacol. 304:107-110, 1978.

Rodin, E.A., Domino, E.F., and Porzak, J.P. The marihuana-induced "social high." Neurological and electroencephalographic concomitants. JAMA 213:1300-1302, 1970.

Rubin, V. and Comitas, L. Ganja in Jamaica: A Medical Anthropological Study of Chronic Marijuana Use. The Hague: Mouton and Co., 1975.

Rumbaugh, C.L., Fang, H.C.H., Wilson, G.H., et al. Cerebral CT findings in drug abuse: Clinical and experimental observations. J. Comput. Assisted Tomography 4:330-334, 1980.

Sipe, J.C. and Moore, R.Y. The lateral hypothalamic area: An ultrastructural analysis. Cell Tiss. Res. 179:177-196, 1977.

Stadnicki, S.W., Schaeppi, U., Rosenkrantz, H., and Braude, M.C. Crude marihuana extract: EEG and behavioral effects of chronic oral administration in rhesus monkeys. Psychopharmacologia 37:225-233, 1974.

Volavka, J., Dornbush, R., Feldstein, S., et al. Marijuana, EEG and behavior. Ann. N.Y. Acad. Sci. 191:206-215, 1971.

Wikler, A. and Lloyd, B. Effect of smoking marijuana cigarettes on cortical electrical activity. Fed. Proc. 4:141, 1945.

5

EFFECTS OF MARIJUANA ON
OTHER BIOLOGICAL SYSTEMS

This chapter covers what little is known about the effects of cannabis on male and female reproduction and endocrine systems, birth defects and teratogenic effects, genetics, the immune system, and body temperature.

MALE REPRODUCTIVE FUNCTION

A variety of studies indicate that marijuana and some of its derivatives have reversible, suppressive effects upon testicular function in animals and men. These have been measured in terms of diminished weights of the prostate gland, seminal vesicles, or testes, and in decreased levels of testosterone (the male hormone) in blood plasma or suppression of spermatogenesis following chronic or acute administration of cannabis or Δ-9-THC. Appropriate observations have indicated that the effects of cannabinoids on the male reproductive tract and on testicular function were completely reversed 1 month after drug withdrawal.

There is no general agreement as to the cause or magnitude of these effects. The major reasons for this lack of agreement relate to major differences in study design, including species studied (man, monkey, or rodent), route of drug administration, and purity of the drug used.

Human Studies

In 1974, a group of 20 men were studied who had used marijuana at least 4 days a week for a minimum of 6 months without the use of other drugs (Kolodny et al., 1974). Plasma testosterone levels in subjects smoking five to nine marijuana cigarettes per week were significantly lower than controls (however, only 2 had levels out of the normal range, i.e., below 400 ng/dl); all but 1 of the men smoking more than 10 marijuana cigarettes per week had testosterone levels below 400 ng/dl. These results suggest that there was a dose-dependent effect of marijuana on testosterone levels. Plasma levels of lutenizing hormone (LH) and follicle-stimulating hormone

94

(FSH), gonadotropins that control the growth of the ovaries or testes and their hormonal activities, were in the normal range; however, in men smoking more than 10 marijuana cigarettes per week, the FSH level was significantly lower than for those who smoked 5 to 10 marijuana cigarettes per week. Because only random samples of blood were obtained for gonadotropic measurements, small but significant changes could have been missed. Levels of prolactin, the female hormone involved in lactation and also present in small quantities in men, were all in the low normal range. In addition, the men who smoked more than 10 marijuana cigarettes per week had significantly lower sperm counts than those who smoked the lesser quantity (26 versus 68 million/ml). These individuals obtained marijuana from a variety of sources, and there was no way to determine whether they were taking other drugs that could lower plasma testosterone.

Later in 1974, another study reported that plasma testosterone levels were not suppressed in 27 men studied in a research ward (Mendelson et al., 1974) These individuals smoked marijuana cigarettes supplied by the federal government. For unexplained reasons, the mean testosterone levels in these individuals were greater than 1,000 ng/dl (higher than the normal mean) before and during the smoking periods. This is in marked contrast to the mean value of 742 ng/dl for nonsmokers in the study of Kolodny et al. mentioned above. There was no report of gonadotropic values or semen analysis in the Mendelson Study.

A study of 16 patients on a metabolic ward who smoked NIDA cigarettes (Hembree et al., 1979) showed that 5 to 6 weeks of high-dose (2 percent) marijuana administration (8-20 cigarettes/day) was associated with a decline in sperm count during the fifth and sixth weeks after initiation of drug exposure. This was preceded by a decrease in sperm motility and an increase in abnormal forms of sperm. Once a week during the study five blood samples were obtained at 15-minute intervals for measurement of testosterone, LH, and FSH. No change in these hormone levels was noted throughout the study (although no values were reported). The relationship in time of these samples to the last previous cigarette was not mentioned, therefore the test would not have excluded a transient decline in hormonal levels after each cigarette. However, because hormonal suppression of spermatogenesis takes longer than 4 weeks and usually is not associated with an increase in the number of abnormal forms and a decrease in motility, the authors concluded that the effect upon the seminiferous tubular epithelium was direct rather than by suppression of gonadotropins. This is the only reported study in man that measured the hour-to-hour fluctuations in gonadotropic levels.

Another study (Coggins et al., 1976) evaluated the health status of 84 marijuana smokers who had used the agent three or more times per week for a minimum of 10 years. Testosterone levels were measured in 38 users and 38 nonusers. The mean levels and ranges were virtually identical. This heterogeneous group of men patients studied in Costa Rica was not recruited for the purpose of studying the pituitary-gonadal axis. No gonadotropic levels or semen samples were studied.

Endocrine function studies are briefly mentioned in a paper by Cohen (1976). Subjects were recruited on the basis of heavy marijuana use and were studied in a metabolic ward. They smoked an average of five marijuana cigarettes per day, which was believed to be the equivalent of 103 mg of Δ-9-THC. During acute administration, mean levels of plasma testosterone declined from 754 to 533 ng/dl over a 3-hour period. After 9 weeks of smoking, plasma testosterone levels had declined from 740 to 509 ng. Plasma LH levels were reported to have fallen after the fourth week; however, no absolute values were given. In addition, no standard errors are given for any of the means presented in this paper. Therefore, it is impossible to evaluate the significance of the reported findings.

In Greece, a population of 47 chronic hashish users was studied. Electron microscope studies of the acrosome, the head of the sperm, showed abnormality in some patients (Issidorides, 1979). It is difficult to evaluate the study because no quantitative data were presented.

Animal Studies

All of the studies mentioned below are substantially different from those of human beings because, with one exception, the active agent (usually Δ-9-THC) was administered intraperitoneally at a dose of 2.5 to 25 mg/kg. Based on calculations given by Cohen (1976), 3 to 6 mg/kg/day would be considered a large dose in human beings.* Also, human beings self-administer the drug over many hours rather than as a single dose.

In castrated rhesus monkeys, plasma LH and FSH fell acutely following acute administration of Δ-9-THC (Smith et al., 1980). During this suppression period, both gonadotropins could be stimulated by lutenizing hormone-releasing factor (LHRF), which causes the release of LH. The effect of Δ-9-THC was to suppress prolactin release, which, in turn, could be stimulated by thyrotropin-releasing hormone (TRH). Studies in other species have tended to confirm these observations in monkeys.

The results are compatible with the hypothesis that the effect of marijuana and its derivatives is on gonadotropic secretion (Harclerode et al., 1979). Testicular cytochrome P-450 (an enzyme) decreased in the rat following 2 to 9 weeks of treatment. The concentrations of this enzyme, plus a variety of other testicular markers, were restored with FSH and LH therapy. The effect of various cannabinoids has been studied on sperm morphology in the mouse (Zimmerman et al., 1979).

---

*Rosenkrantz (1981) considers 0.6-3.0 mg/kg by inhalation and 1.8-9.0 mg/kg orally to be large doses in human beings. For the monkey, 1.8-9.0 mg/kg by inhalation and 5-27 mg/kg orally would be considered a high dose. (These concentrations are equivalent to six cigarettes/day.)

Mice were given five daily intraperitoneal injections of Δ-9-THC, cannabidiol, or cannabinol at doses approaching or exceeding the LD_{50} (the dose necessary to kill 50 percent of the animals). Thirty-five days after the last treatment, animals were killed and sperm were evaluated by scanning electron microscopy. Control animals had 1.5 percent abnormal forms. Animals that received LD_{50} doses of the various derivatives had 2.4 to 5.0 percent abnormal forms.

Only a few studies have examined the effects of cannabis on spermatogenesis (Huang et al., 1979). Marijuana was administered to rats in a smoke machine. After 30 days of exposure, marijuana smoke lowered the sperm counts in animals significantly, as did cannabinoid-free smoke. By 75 days, however, only the marijuana smoke group maintained a low sperm count. In the marijuana-treated group, there was an increased number of abnormal forms, particularly with an increase in dissociation of sperm heads and tails. In the discussion of this paper, the authors reported elevated serum FSH levels following marijuana exposure, but did not present data. They concluded that marijuana has a direct effect on the testis. A variety of in vitro studies support this suggestion (Jakubovic et al., 1977, 1979).

Marijuana and its derivatives also have been shown to be antiandrogenic (antagonistic to male hormones) (Purohit et al., 1980). Several constituents, including Δ-9-THC, can bind to the receptor for androgen. Marijuana also has been demonstrated to be estrogenic (like female sex hormones) in vivo, and recent studies suggest that these effects may be mediated via the estrogen receptor. These observations have been disputed by others (reviewed by Purohit et al., 1980). The ability to inhibit or mimic the action of sex steroids provides one mechanism by which these agents can produce their effects. There obviously are many others.

FEMALE REPRODUCTIVE FUNCTION

The effect of cannabis on female reproduction has been studied in rats, mice, rabbits, and monkeys. The work in rhesus monkeys is of particular importance, because of the similarity in the menstrual cycle among primate species, including human beings.

Human Studies

There is only one study reported on the effects of marijuana on reproductive function in women. The work has appeared in print as a report of the proceedings of a 1978 symposium held in Mexico City (Bauman et al., 1979) and as part of the congressional record subsequent to testimony before a Senate committee hearing (Bauman, 1980). These publications do not provide details on methodology or on individual hormone values. Differences between the control and experimental groups, recognized by the investigators, could be of

98

importance; alcohol use, for example, was more frequent in the
marijuana-using group. The study attempted to establish the endocrine
(hormonal) profile and menstrual patterns of women who used marijuana
on a chronic and frequent basis. Twenty-six women who used it at
least three times a week for 6 months were compared with 17 women who
had never used the substance. The number of cycles studied for each
variable investigated is not clear from the publications. This
difficulty notwithstanding, the report reveals no difference in plasma
levels of LH and FSH between the two groups and no change in peaks
and basal values of the female hormones estradiol or progesterone,
the critical hormone levels controlling the process of ovulation. It
would be expected that no major difference was found in the incidence
of anovulatory cycles between the two groups. By combining anovulation and shortened luteal phase, however, the authors report a
statistically significant difference in the marijuana-using group,
which could be clinically important in causing subfertility. This
evidence is, at best, only suggestive. The observation that
testosterone levels in marijuana-using women are elevated is
difficult to interpret in terms of clinical significance; apparently,
the subjects did not report episodes of acne, abnormal hairiness, or
other testosterone-dependent side-effects. According to the authors,
serum prolactin levels are lower in marijuana users than in controls.
The implications of this observation for fertility, lactation, or the
development of breast cancer are not clear.

The absence of other studies on users of marijuana makes it
difficult to draw conclusions on the implications of the data cited
above. Several of the effects noted are different from the more
extensive and experimentally controlled observations in rhesus
monkeys and other laboratory animals. This situation calls attention
to the urgent need for more comprehensive endocrine and gynecologic
investigations of women who use marijuana.

Animal Studies

Administration of crude marijuana extract to rats or mice resulted
generally in suppression of ovarian function and in various aspects
of estrogen activity, such as uterine metabolism, weight, glycogen
content, and levels of RNA and sialic acid (Chakravarty et al., 1975;
Dixit et al., 1975).

The administration of crude marijuana extract for 30 days to rats
and mice abolished the estrus cycle and caused a significant reduction
in the size of the ovaries and in some primordial ova (Dixit et al.,
1975). Intraperitoneal administration of Δ-9-THC to rats,
appropriately timed, has also been reported to block ovulation (Nir
et al., 1973). This effect of Δ-9-THC was exerted by suppressing
the characteristic preovulatory surge of plasma LH. Other
investigators have reported suppression also of plasma FSH and
prolactin when Δ-9-THC is given just before ovulation (Ayalon et
al., 1977). The substance was found to depress plasma concentration
of LH in ovariectomized rats (Marks, 1973; Tyrey, 1978, 1980) and

rhesus monkeys (Besch et al., 1977). Asch et al. (1979) also showed in the rabbit, a reflex ovulator, that a precoital single dose of Δ-9-THC blocks the postcoital LH surge and ovulation.

Administration of LHRF was able to bring about the release of LH in Δ-9-THC treated rats and rhesus monkeys (Smith et al., 1979). These results indicate a direct effect of cannabinoids at the level of the hypothalamus, part of brain important in reproductive hormone regulation. The ovulation-blocking effect of the cannabinoids was further investigated by Cordova et al. (1980). Natural and chemically modified cannabinoids blocked ovulation in rats.

Administration of Δ-9-THC to rhesus monkeys during the follicular phase resulted in prolonged periods of amennorhea (absence or abnormal stoppage of the menstrual flow), absence of midcycle LH surge, and progesterone levels characteristic of anovulation (Asch et al., 1981).

BIRTH DEFECTS AND TERATOGENICITY

Because Δ-9-THC crosses the placenta it is a potential teratogen, an agent that causes defects in the developing embryo. This effect could occur in either of two ways: (1) exposure to cannabis prior to conception could harm the sex cells (the ova and sperm), or (2) the fetus could be harmed directly during organogenesis. In addition, Δ-9-THC can be secreted in breast milk and, therefore, can be toxic postnatally.

Human Studies

The evidence for teratogenicity in human beings is very difficult to interpret. Although there is widespread use of marijuana in young women of reproductive age, there is no evidence yet of any teratogenic effects of high frequency or consistent association with the drug. There are isolated reports of congenital anomalies in the offspring of marijuana users, but there is no evidence that they occurred more often in users than in nonusers and in those cases there was coincident use of other drugs. Subtle development effects in offspring, such as nervous system abnormalities, and reductions in birth weight and height may indeed exist (Finnegan, 1980; Fried, 1980; Hingson et al., in press). Additional carefully designed, prospective studies should provide valuable information in this area.

Animal Studies

Crude marijuana extract and Δ-9-THC are teratogenic at certain doses in animals.*

---

*Bibliography available upon request from the Institute of Medicine, National Academy of Sciences.

One study reported that subcutaneous injection of pregnant hamsters and rabbits with various doses of crude marijuana extract caused malformations of the brain, spinal cord, forelimb, and liver, as well as edema of the head and spinal region in developing embryos (Gerber and Schramm, 1969). In hamsters, significant embryocidal and growth retardation effects also were noted. It was concluded that doses greater than 200 mg/kg in hamsters and 250 mg/kg in rabbits were teratogenic. Caution in interpreting these findings must be exercised because the teratogenic effects may be caused by any combination of constituents of the cannabis extract.

In a study of mice, the teratological effects of Δ-9-THC were evaluated for doses ranging from 3.0 to 400 mg/kg by various routes of administration--intravenous, subcutaneous, and intragastric (Joneja, 1976). Significant fetal growth retardation was induced at higher dose levels and by some routes of administration. For example, a high dose of 400 mg/kg was significantly teratogenic by the intragastric route; 12.1 percent of the live fetuses were malformed.

In a study of female monkeys given an oral dose of 2.4 mg/kg Δ-9-THC for 1 to 4 years, a nonspecific pattern of reproductive difficulties was observed characteristic of "high-risk" pregnancies, including a high rate of offspring loss during pregnancy or in the early postnatal period (Sassenrath et al., 1979).

GENETIC EFFECTS

The potential genetic effects of marijuana are of major concern because of its prevalent use by young people in their reproductive years (see Chapter 2). Although there is a growing amount of evidence that drugs can induce mutations, and an improving ability to use toxicological methods to evaluate agents for their mutagenic potential (such as the Ames test, which detects changes or damages in the genetic material), the available information on the genetic hazards or even on the potential genetic hazards of the use of marijuana is extremely limited.

Mutagenicity

Elsewhere in this report (Chapter 3) the scientific evidence that marijuana smoke and tar are mutagenic has been discussed. Lung explants of mice and human fibroblast cultures exposed to fresh smoke showed abnormalities of cell division, as well as changes in chromosome structure and in DNA synthesis (Leuchtenberger and Leuchtenberger, 1971; Leuchtenberger, et al., 1973a,b). Moreover, extracts and smoke condensates of marijuana are mutagenic when evaluated by the Ames test (Busch et al., 1979; Seid and Wei, 1979; Wehner et al., 1980). Animal studies on rodents painted with marijuana tar, three times weekly for 1 year, resulted in skin papillomas, carcinomas, and fibrosarcomas (Hoffmann et al., 1975).

However, extensive testing with Δ-9-THC using three established tests for mutagenesis failed to detect any mutagenic effect, or any effect as an inhibitor of DNA repair (Legator et al., 1976; Glatt et al., 1979; Zimmerman et al., 1978).

Cytogenetic Effects

The numbers and kinds of chromosomes (structures in a cell nucleus that contain and transmit genetic information carried in DNA) are highly characteristic for a given species. Structural variation and changes in numbers of chromosomes may be evidence for genetic damage produced by drugs and other chemical agents. Unfortunately, the literature on the effects of marijuana on chromosomes is limited and conflicting. Studies suggesting that marijuana probably does not break chromosomes are fairly conclusive. There is less evidence that marijuana may produce aneuploidy (abnormal numbers of chromosomes) in some daughter cells during cell division.

Does marijuana cause chromosome breaks? The weight of the evidence from in vitro cultures of human cells and from in vivo animal and human studies is that neither marijuana nor Δ-9-THC causes chromosome breaks.

In Vitro and Animal Studies

Cultures of human leukocytes, exposed to different concentrations of Δ-9-THC, showed no increase in the incidence of chromosome breaks or gaps when compared to controls (Stenchever and Allen, 1972). Studies of golden hamsters given subcutaneous injections for 10 days of marijuana extract distillate containing 17.1 percent Δ-9-THC (Nicholson et al., 1973), and of beagle dogs trained to smoke high doses of marijuana (3 g/day/week for 30 months), showed no significant differences in chromosome gaps or breaks when compared with control groups (Genest et al., 1976).

Human Studies

Cytogenetic analysis of chromosomes from peripheral blood leukocytes and cultures of subjects exposed to marijuana smoking, marijuana extract, or synthetic Δ-9-THC revealed no increase in chromosome breakage attributable to these compounds (Nichols et al., 1974; Matsuyama, 1976; Morishima et al., 1979). Doses ranged from 20 mg Δ-9-THC per day to 12-16 marijuana cigarettes per day. Studies that have reported chromosome breaks or gaps in cell cultures of users of marijuana have largely been carried out on multiple drug users, and the breaks and gaps may be due to other factors associated with a life of heavy drug use (Gilmour et al., 1971; Herha and Obe, 1974). However, in a retrospective study on college students, chromosome breaks were found in blood cultures of 49 light (one or less exposure per week) and heavy (more than two exposures per week) users of marijuana (Stenchever et al., 1974). One problem in this study is the poor dose characterization. Furthermore, the increase in the numbers of breaks in both light and heavy users of marijuana was not dose-related; the same frequency of breaks was observed in both groups. Although the evidence is inconclusive, it suggests that marijuana does not cause chromosome breaks.

Does marijuana interfere with cell division and chromosome segregation, thereby resulting in abnormal numbers of chromosomes? There is conflicting evidence in the literature. On the one hand, no significant effects of marijuana smoke or Δ-9-THC on chromosome complement have been reported using the micronuclei test in mice or in cytogenetic studies in dogs (Genest et al., 1976; Legator et al., 1976). On the other hand, more extensive studies have demonstrated aneuploidy resulting from in vitro exposure of cells to marijuana as well as in vivo studies of animals and human beings.

In Vitro and Animal Studies

Exposure of mouse lung and adult human lung tissue culture to marijuana smoke in vitro resulted in abnormal cell proliferation and abnormalities in DNA content (Leuchtenberger and Leuchtenberger, 1971; Leuchtenberger, et al., 1973b). Addition of Δ-9-THC and olivetol, a compound with a ring structure similar to cannabinoids, to normal human leukocyte cultures induced hypodiploidy (defined as metaphase nuclei with a chromosome complement of less than 30 chromosomes--a normal human cell contains 46 chromosomes) (Morishima et al., 1976). Hybrid mice treated for 5 consecutive days with Δ-9-THC, cannabinol, and cannabidiol at a dose of 10 mg/kg had a three- to fivefold increase of micronuclei over controls. The number of micronuclei increased with increasing Δ-9-THC dosage. Examination of bone marrow mitosis in these same mice showed a five- to sevenfold increase in chromosome number aberrations during metaphase (Zimmerman and Raj, 1980).

Human Studies

Studies of lymphocytes cultured from human marijuana smokers defined either as "moderate" users (at least one marijuana cigarette per week, range 1-10 for a minimum of two years) or "heavy" users (more than three times per week) all of whom consumed between 12.9 and 15.3 marijuana cigarettes per day during the experiment, turned up a significantly larger number of cells with less than 30 chromosomes than would be found in normal control cultures (Morishima et al., 1979). These positive findings suggest that marijuana may affect chromosome segregation during cell division and result in cells with fewer than the normal number of chromosomes. What these findings mean in terms of risk for abnormalities in offspring or possible disease is not known. Findings in lymphocyte cultures may not be relevant to what is happening in the germ cells (sex cells).

THE IMMUNE SYSTEM

The immune system functions in protecting the body against viruses, bacteria, and other infections. It also plays a major role in preventing the growth and dissemination of cancerous cells.

There have been reports that cannabis is immunogenic, capable of activating components in the immune system. These components include such cells as lymphocytes, some of which produce antibodies in response to invasion by a foreign agent, and macrophages, which can be stimulated by inflammation to ingest invaders.

Human Studies

There have been reports that cannabis interferes with components in the immune system in man. Antibodies will develop in response to marijuana in some people, along with an allergic response, while others develop antibodies without apparent allergic reaction (Liskow et al., 1971; Shapiro et al., 1974, 1976; Lewis and Slavin, 1975). However, the studies reporting these effects were not designed to determine which components of the marijuana are immunogenic and which are allergenic.

Studies of various aspects of the immune system in persons who were chronic users of marijuana have indicated mild decreases in activity of one or another component of the system; however, other investigators have noted no changes outside of the normal range (Gupta et al., 1974; Petersen et al., 1975, 1976; White et al., 1975; Lau et al., 1976; Rachelefsky et al., 1976; Silverstein and Lessin, 1976; Cushman and Khurana, 1977; McDonough et al., 1980). These apparent inconsistencies may stem from the variability in the amount of marijuana consumed among users in different studies and the differences in the immune system assays. Hashish, as distinct from marijuana, was shown to have a slight temporary stimulatory effect on the immune system (Kaklamani et al., 1978; Kalofoutis et al., 1978).

Animal Studies

A number of studies have shown that Δ-9-THC and other cannabinoids induce immunological defects in rodents (Petersen and Lemberger, 1976; Lefkowitz and Klager, 1978, Lefkowitz et al., 1978; Preuss and Lefkowitz, 1978). The doses varied from 5 to 25 mg/kg (intraperitoneally) to 100 mg/kg (orally). At the higher doses there was a diminution of immune response, as measured by standard immunological assays. Delta-9-THC had the same effects on cells grown in vitro. Other cannabinoids also have been tested for their effects. Cannabinol, Δ-8-THC, and 1-methyl-Δ-8-THC had the same immunosuppressive effects as Δ-9-THC, but cannabidiol had no immunosuppressive effect. Immunizing rabbits with Δ-9-THC resulted in the production of antibodies (Chiarotti et al., 1980).

BODY TEMPERATURE

Regulation of body temperature is a complex process that can be influenced by drugs. In several species of animals, Δ-9-THC produces a lowering of body temperature (hypothermia). The effect is seen when animals are housed at normal room temperatures, and it is greater with colder ambient temperatures (Pertwee and Travendale, 1979). Marijuana apparently causes a decrease in heat production for reasons that are unclear.

In experiments with human subjects, marijuana has produced little or no change in body temperature when given in a cool environment (Beaconsfield et al., 1972; Hanna et al., 1976). In a hot environment (40°C) marijuana caused inhibition of sweating and a consistent rise in body temperature (Jones et al., 1980). Thus, there is evidence that marijuana does interfere with temperature regulation, although there is no currently known clinical significance to this finding.

Cannabis appears to interfere with temperature regulation, but the clinical significance is unknown.

SUMMARY

Male Reproductive Function

In animals, marijuana and its derivatives can acutely lower gonadotropic secretion when administered intraperitoneally. There is also some evidence in animals to suggest that these agents can directly affect the seminiferous tubule. In man, sperm number and motility are decreased during chronic marijuana use. From the available studies, it appears this was due to a direct effect of the cannabinoids either on the seminiferous tubular epithelium or the epididymal sperm. Due to conflicting and incomplete evidence, it is not possible to conclude at the present time whether marijuana smoking has a significant effect upon gonadotropic and testosterone concentrations in humans. Whether the decrease in sperm number or motility has any effect on fertility is not known.

Female Reproductive Function

There is only one study of human beings that attempts to establish the endocrine profile and menstrual patterns of women who used marijuana on a chronic and frequent basis. By combining categories of anovulation and shortened luteal phase, a statistically significant difference was noticed in the marijuana using group. It is not known if this leads to problems with fertility or lactation, or if it leads to cancer of the reproductive organs.

Animal studies have shown that Δ-9-THC lowers the serum gonadotropic levels. It is unknown if there is a direct effect on the reproductive tissues, particularly under prolonged use of cannabis products.

Birth Defects and Teratogencity

Cannabis is teratogenic at high doses in animals. There is no
evidence of obvious teratogenicity or structural defects in the
offspring of human users. But the data are not adequate to reveal a
long-range functional impairment or a very low level of teratogenicity if one is present. It may be impossible to identify a
distinct role for cannabis in the production of subtle effects in
offspring, because of the confounding influences of malnutrition,
smoking, and alcohol.

Genetic Effects

Marijuana and Δ-9-THC do not appear to break chromosomes, although
there is some conflicting evidence on this point. Multiple drug use
seems to be correlated with an increase in the numbers of gaps and
breaks in the genetic material. Furthermore, marijuana may affect
chromosome segregation during cell division, resulting in abnormal
numbers of chromosomes in daughter cells. While these conflicting
results are worrisome, their clinical significance is not known.
Further investigations, especially controlled prospective studies, of
human beings are needed.

The Immune System

The data from animal studies suggest that Δ-9-THC and some of its
analogues have a mild, transient, immunosuppressant effect in both _in
vitro_ and _in vivo_ systems; the effects are mild compared with known
immunosuppressant drugs. The studies in human beings are contradictory; some demonstrated mild, immunosuppressive effects, but others,
using the same or similar methods, did not find any differences in
the immune system between normals and chronic marijuana smokers. At
the present time, there have been no human or animal studies that
have determined if marijuana smokers are more prone to infections or
other diseases. Because of the widespread use of marijuana, even
weak immunosuppressive effects are a concern. Since further research
may not demonstrate definitive findings, immunologic effects should
be studied along with other variables in a larger investigation. If
marijuana is to be used on immunosuppressed patients (for example,
for antiemetic purposes during cancer chemotherapy), even minor
additional suppression might be dangerous.

RECOMMENDATIONS FOR RESEARCH

The committee recommends the following types of studies.

• Further observations should be made regarding the relation
of marijuana use to reproductive defects in human beings, especially

on young users whose reproductive biology is undergoing rapid change. The principal need is for assessment of endocrine profiles and semen analysis in male users versus nonusers, with adequate control of confounding variables--for example, diet, alcohol, other drug use. In women, the principal need is for more data on endocrine and menstrual patterns in users versus nonusers, with particular attention to the length of cycles, the presence or absence of ovulation, and the existence or absence of subfertility. More studies are needed to detect subtle, low-frequency, or cumulative effects on reproductive function in long-term, heavy users.

• Although routine testing of teratogenicity in human beings is not recommended at this time, the collection of precise epidemiologic information on the outcome of human pregnancy in marijuana users is of great importance and must be carefully controlled.

• There are no good animal models for studying the effects of smoking marijuana, but cytogenetic studies in animals after exposure to Δ-9-THC by other routes than smoking would be of some value. The most relevant studies still would be in vivo human studies.

• Marijuana has been found to have mild immunological effects in a variety of test systems, but studies of its influence on the body's immune defense against microorganisms are lacking and need to be conducted.

• Critical experiments are needed to test the hypothesis that Δ-9-THC causes disruption of thermoregulatory effector responses rather than an alteration of the level of thermoregulation.

• Inherited variation in the way some drugs are metabolized is widely recognized. This type of variation must be evaluated in respect to susceptibility to marijuana.

REFERENCES

Asch, R.H., Fernandez, E.O., Smith, C.G., and Pauerstein, C.J. Precoital single doses of Δ-9-tetrahydrocannabinol block ovulation in the rabbit. Fertil. Steril. 31:331-334, 1979.

Asch, R.H., Smith, C.G., Siler-Khodr, T.M., and Pauerstein, C.J. Effects of Δ-9-tetrahydrocannabinol during the follicular phase of the Rhesus monkey (Macaca mulatta). J. Clin. Endocrin. Metab. 52:50-55, 1981.

Ayalon, D., Nir, I., Cordova, T., Bauminger, S., et al. Acute effect of Δ-1-tetrahydrocannabinol on the hypothalamo-pituitary-ovarian axis in the rat. Neuroendocrinology 23:31-42, 1977.

Bauman, J. Marijuana and the female reproductive system, pp. 85-88. Testimony before the Subcommittee on Criminal Justice of the Committee on the Judiciary, U.S. Senate, "Health Consequences of Marihuana Use," January 16-17, 1980. Washington, DC: U.S. Government Printing Office, 1980.

Bauman, J.E., Kolodny, R.C., Dornbusch, R.L., and Webster, S.K. Efectos endocrinos del uso cronico de la mariguana en mujeres, pp. 85-97. In Simposio Internacional Sobre Actualizacion en Mariguana, Volume 10. Tlalpan, Mexico, July 1979.

Beaconsfield, P., Ginsburg, J., and Rainsbury, R. Marihuana smoking: Cardiovascular effects in man and possible mechanisms. N. Engl. J. Med. 287:209-212, 1972.

Besch, N.F., Smith, C.G., Besch, P.K., and Kaufman, R.H. The effect of marihuana (delta-9-tetrahydrocannabinol) on the secretion of lutenizing hormone in ovariectomized Rhesus monkey. Am. J. Obstet. Gynecol. 128:635-642, 1977.

Busch, F.W., Seid, D.A., and Wei, E.T. Mutagenic activity of marihuana smoke condensates. Cancer Lett. 6:319-324, 1979.

Chakravarty, I., Sengupta, D., Bhattacharyya, P., and Ghosh, J.J. Effect of treatment with cannabis extract on the water and glycogen contents of the uterus in normal and estradiol-treated prepubertal rats. Toxicol. Appl. Pharmacol. 34:513-516, 1975.

Chiarotti, M., Giusti, G.V., and Vigevani, F. In vivo and in vitro properties of anti-delta-9-tetrahydrocannabinol antibody. Drug Alcohol Dependence 5:231-233, 1980.

Coggins, W.J., Swenson, E.W., Dawson, W.W., et al. Health status of chronic heavy cannabis users. Ann. N.Y. Acad. Sci. 282:148-161, 1976.

Cohen, S. The 94-day cannabis study. Ann. N.Y. Acad. Sci. 282:211-220, 1976.

Cordova, T., Ayalon, D., Lander, N., et al. The ovulation blocking effect of cannabinoids: Structure-activity relationships. Psychoneuroendocrinology 5:53-62, 1980.

Cottrell, J.C., Sohn, S.S., and Vogel, W.H. Toxic effects of marihuana tar on mouse skin. Arch. Environ. Health 26:277-278, 1973.

Cushman, P. and Khurana, R. A controlled cycle of tetrahydro-cannabinol smoking: T and B cell rosette formation. Life Sci. 20:971-979, 1977.

Dixit, V.P., Arya, M., and Lohiya, N.K. The effect of chronically administered cannabis extract on the female genital tract of mice and rats. Endokrinologie 66:365-368, 1975.

Finnegan, L.P. Pulmonary problems encountered by the infant of the drug-dependent mother. Clin. Chest Med. 1:311-325, 1980.

Fried, P.A. Marihuana use by pregnant women: Neurobehavioral effects in neonates. Drug Alcohol Dependence 6:415-424, 1980.

Genest, P., Huy, N.D., and Roy, P.D. Toxicity study of marijuana in dogs: Effects on the mitotic index and chromosomes. Res. Commun. Psychol. Psychiatr. Behav. 1:83-290, 1976.

Gerber, W.F. and Schramm, L.C. Effect of marihuana extract on fetal hamsters and rabbits. Toxicol. Appl. Pharmacol. 14:276-282, 1969.

Gilmour, D.G., Bloom, A.D., Lele, K.P., et al. Chromosomal aberrations in users of psychoactive drugs. Arch. Gen. Psychiatry 24:268-272, 1971.

Glatt, H., Ohlsson, A., Agurell, S., and Oesch, F. Delta-1-tetrahydrocannabinol and 1-alpha, 2-alpha-epoxyhexahydro-cannabinol: Mutagenicity investigation in the Ames test. Mutat. Res. 66:329-335, 1979.

Gupta, S., Grieco, M.H., and Cushman, P. Impairment of rosette-forming T-lymphocytes in chronic marihuana smokers. N. Engl. J. Med. 291:874-877, 1974.

Hanna, J.M., Strauss, R.H., Itagaki, B., et al. Marijuana smoking and cold tolerance in man. Aviation, Space, and Environmental Medicine 47:634-639, 1976.

Harclerode, J., Nyquist, S.E., Nazar, B., and Lowe, D. Effects of cannabis on sex hormones and testicular enzymes of the rodent, pp. 395-405. In Nahas, G.G. and Paton, W.D.M. (eds.) Marihuana: Biological Effects. Analysis, Metabolism, Cellular Responses, Reproduction and Brain. Oxford: Pergamon Press, 1979.

Hembree, W.C., Nahas, G.G., Zeidenberg, P., and Huang, H.F.S. Changes in human spermatozoa associated with high dose marihuana smoking, pp. 429-439. In Nahas, G.G. and Paton, W.D.M. (eds.) Marihuana: Biological Effects. Analysis, Metabolism, Cellular Responses, Reproduction and Brain. Oxford: Pergamon Press, 1979.

Herha, J. and Obe, G. Chromosomal damage in chronical users of cannabis in vivo investigation with two-day leukocyte cultures. Pharmakopsychiat. 7:328-337, 1974.

Hingson, R., Alpert, J.J., Day, N. et al. Effects of maternal drinking and marijuana use on fetal growth and development. J. Pediatr. (in press).

Hoffmann, D., Brunnemann, K.D., Gori, G.B., and Wynder, E.L. On the carcinogenicity of marijuana smoke, pp. 63-81. In Runeckles, V.C. (ed.) Recent Advances in Phytochemistry. New York: Plenum Publishing Corporation, 1975.

Huang, H.F.S., Nahas, G.G., and Hembree, W.C. Effects of marihuana inhalation on spermatogenesis of the rat, pp. 419-427. In Nahas, G.G. and Paton, W.D.M. (eds.) Marihuana: Biological Effects. Analysis, Metabolism, Cellular Responses, Reproduction and Brain. Oxford: Pergamon Press, 1979.

Issidorides, M.R. Observations in chronic hashish users: Nuclear aberrations in blood and sperm and abnormal acrosomes in spermatozoa, pp. 377-388. In Nahas, G.G. and Paton, W.D.M. (eds.) Marihuana: Biological Effects. Analysis, Metabolism, Cellular Responses, Reproduction and Brain. Oxford: Pergamon Press, 1979.

Jakubovic, A. and McGeer, P.L. Biochemical changes in rat testicular cells in vitro produced by cannabinoids and alcohol: Metabolism and incorporation of labeled glucose, amino acids, and nucleic acid precursors. Toxicol. Appl. Pharmacol. 41:473-486, 1977.

Jakubovic, A., McGeer, E.G., and McGeer, P.L. Effects of cannabinoids on testosterone and protein synthesis in rat testis Leydig cells in vitro. Molec. Cell. Endocrinol. 15:41-50, 1979.

Joneja, M.G. A study of teratological effects of intravenous, subcutaneous, and intragastric administration of Δ-9-tetrahydrocannabinol in mice. Toxicol. Appl. Pharmacol. 36:151-162, 1976.

Jones, E.P., Manno, J.E., Brown, R.D., et al. Tachycardia in rats following intracerebroventricular (ICV) administration of Δ-9-tetrahydrocannabinol (THC). Fed. Proc. Fed. Am. Soc. Exp. Biol. 39:848, 1980.

Kaklamani, E., Trichopoulos, D., Koutselinis, A., et al. Hashish smoking and T-lymphocytes. Arch. Toxicol. 40:97-101, 1978.

Kalofoutis, A., Koutselinis, A., Dionyssiou-Asteriou, A., and Miras, C. The significance of lymphocyte lipid changes after smoking hashish. Acta Pharmacol. Toxicol. 43:81-85, 1978.

Kolodny, R.C., Masters, W.H., Kolodner, R.M., and Toro, G. Depression of plasma testosterone levels after chronic intensive marijuana use. N. Engl. J. Med. 290:872-874, 1974.

Lau, R.J., Tubergen, D.G., Barr, M., and Domino, E.F. Phytohemagglutinin-induced lymphocyte transformation in humans receiving delta-9-tetrahydrocannabinol. Science 192:805-807, 1976.

Lefkowitz, S.S. and Klager, K. Effect of delta-9-tetrahydro-cannabinol on in vitro sensitization of mouse splenic lymphocytes. Immunol. Commun. 7:557-566, 1978.

Lefkowitz, S.S., Klager, K., Nemeth, D., and Pruess, M. Immuno-suppression of mice by delta-9-tetrahydrocannabinol. Res. Commun. Chem. Pathol. Pharmacol. 19:101-107, 1978.

Legator, M.S., Weber, E., Connor, T., and Stoeckel, M. Failure to detect mutagenic effects of Δ-9-tetrahydrocannabinol in the dominant lethal test, host-mediated assay, blood-urine studies, and cytogenetic evaluation with mice, pp. 699-709. In Braude, M.C. and Szara, S. (eds.) Pharmacology of Marihuana. New York: Raven Press, 1976.

Leuchtenberger, C. and Leuchtenberger, R. Morphological and cytochemical effects of marijuana cigarette smoke on epithelioid cells of lung explants from mice. Nature 234:227-229, 1971.

Leuchtenberger, C., Leuchtenberger, R., and Schneider, A. Effects of marijuana and tobacco smoke on human lung physiology. Nature 241:137-139, 1973a.

Leuchtenberger, C., Leuchtengerger, R., Ritter, U., and Inui, N. Effects of marijuana and tobacco smoke on DNA and chromosomal complement in human lung explants. Nature 242:403-404, 1973b.

Lewis, C.R. and Slavin, R.G. Allergy to marijuana: A clinical and skin-testing study. J. Allergy Clin. Immunol. 55:131-132, 1975.

Liskow, B., Liss, J.L., and Parker, C.W. Allergy to marihuana. Ann. Intern. Med. 75:571-573, 1971.

Marks, B.H. Δ-1-tetrahydrocannabinol and luteinizing hormone secretion. Prog. Brain Res. 39:331-338, 1973.

Matsuyama, S.S., Jarvik, L.F., Fu, T., and Yen, F. Chromosome studies before and after supervised marijuana smoking, pp. 723-729. In Braude, M.C. and Szara, S. (eds.) Pharmacology of Marihuana. New York: Raven Press, 1976.

McDonough, R.J., Madden, J.J., Falek, A., et al. Alteration of T and null lymphocyte frequencies in the peripheral blood of human opiate addicts: In vivo evidence for opiate receptor sites on T lymphocytes. J. Immunol. 125:2539-2543, 1980.

Mendelson, J.H., Kuehnle, J., Ellingboe, J., and Babor, T.F. Plasma testosterone levels before, during and after chronic marihuana smoking. N. Engl. J. Med. 291:1051-1055, 1974.

Morishima, A., Milstein, M., Henrich, R.T., and Nahas, G.G. Effects of marihuana smoking, cannabinoids, and olivetol on replication of human lymphocytes: Formation of micronuclei, pp. 711-722. In Braude, M.C. and Szara, S. (eds.) Pharmacology of Marihuana. New York: Raven Press, 1976.

Morishima, A., Henrich, R.T., Jayaraman, J., and Nahas, G.G. Hypoploid metaphases in cultured lymphocytes of marihuana smokers, pp. 371-376. In Nahas, G.G. and Paton, W.D.M. (eds.) Marihuana: Biological Effects. Analysis, Metabolism, Cellular Responses, Reproduction and Brain. Oxford: Pergamon Press, 1979.

Nichols, W.W., Miller, R.C., Heneen, W. et al. Cytogenetic studies on human subjects receiving marihuana and Δ-9-tetrahydrocannabinol. Mutat. Res. 26:413-417, 1974.

Nicholson, M.T., Pace, H.B., and Davis, W.M. Effects of marihuana and lysergic acid diethylamide on leukocyte chromosomes of the golden hamster. Res. Commun. Chem. Pathol. Pharmacol. 6:427-434, 1973.

Nir, I., Ayalon, D., Tsafriri, A. et al. Suppression of the cyclic surge of luteinizing hormone secretion and of ovulation in the rat by Δ-1-tetrahydrocannabinol. Nature 243:470-471, 1973.

Pertwee, R.G. and Tavendale, R. Effects of Δ-9-tetrahydrocannabinol, 2.4-dinitrophenol and pentolinium tartrate on behavioral thermoregulation in mice. Br. J. Pharmacol. 66:39-50, 1979.

Petersen, B.H., Lemberger, L., Graham, J., and Dalton, B. Alterations in the cellular-mediated immune responsiveness of chronic marihuana smokers. Psychopharmacol. Commun. 1:67-74, 1975.

Petersen, B.H., Graham, J., and Lemberger, L. Marihuana, tetrahydrocannabinol and T-cell function. Life Sci. 19:395-400, 1976.

Petersen, B.H. and Lemberger, L. Effect of delta-9-tetrahydrocannabinol administration of antibody production in mice. Fed. Proc. 35:333, 1976.

Pruess, M.M. and Lefkowitz, S.S. Influence of maturity on immunosuppression by delta-9-tetrahydrocannabinol. Proc. Soc. Exp. Biol. Med. 158:350-353, 1978.

Purohit, V., Ahluwahlia, B.S., and Vigersky, R.A. Marihuana inhibits dihydrotestosterone binding to the androgen receptor. Endocrinology 107:848-850, 1980.

Rachelefsky, G.S., Opelz, G., Mickey, M.R., et al. Intact humoral and cell-mediated immunity in chronic marijuana smoking. J. Allergy Clin. Immunol. 58:483-490, 1976.

Rosenkrantz, H. In Report of an Addiction Research Foundation/World Health Organization (ARF/WHO) Scientific Meeting on Adverse Health of Behavioral Consequences of Marijuana Use. ARF/WHO, Toronto, 1981.

Sassenrath, E.N., Banovitz, C.A., and Chapman, L.F. Tolerance and reproductive deficit in primates chronically drugged with Δ-9-THC. Pharmacologist 21:201, 1979.

Seid, D.A. and Wei, E.T. Mutagenic activity of marihuana smoke condensates. Pharmacologist 21:204, 1979.

Shapiro, C.M., Orlina, A.R., Unger, P., and Billings, A.A. Antibody response to cannabis. JAMA 230:81-82, 1974.

Shapiro, C.M., Orlina, A.R., Unger, P.J., et al. Marihuana-induced antibody response. J. Lab. Clin. Med. 88:194-201, 1976.

Silverstein, M.J. and Lessin P. 2,4-dinitrochlorobenzene skin testing in chronic marihuana users, pp. 199-203. In Braude, M.C. and Szara, S. (eds.) Pharmacology of Marihuana New York: Raven Press, 1976.

Smith, C.G., Besch, N.F., Smith, R.G., and Besch, P.K. Effect of tetrahydrocannabinol on the hypothalamic-pituitary axis in the ovariectomized Rhesus monkey. Fertil. Steril. 31:335-339, 1979.

Smith, C.G., Besch, N.F., and Asch, R.H. Effects of marihuana on the reproductive system, pp. 273-294. In Thomas, J.A. and Singhal, R.L. (eds.) Advances in Sex Hormone Research Baltimore: Urban and Schwarzenberg, 1980.

Stenchever, M.A. and Allen, M. The effect of delta-9-tetrahydrocannabinol on the chromosomes of human lymphocytes in vitro. Am. J. Obstet. Gynecol. 114:819-821, 1972.

Stenchever, M.A., Kunysz, T.J., and Allen, M.A. Chromosome breakage in users of marihuana. Am. J. Obstet. Gynecol. 118:106-113, 1974.

Tyrey, L. Δ-9-Tetrahydrocannabinol suppression of episodic luteinizing hormone secretion in the ovariectomized rat. Endocrinology 102:1808-1814, 1978.

Tyre, L. Δ-9-Tetrahydrocannabinol: A potent inhibitor of episodic luteinizing hormone secretion. J. Pharmacol. Exp. Ther. 213:306-308, 1980.

Wehner, F.C., Van Rensburg, S.J., and Thiel, P.G. Mutagenicity of marijuana and transkei tobacco smoke condensates in the salmonella/microsome assay. Mutat. Res. 77:135-142, 1980.

White, S.C., Brin, S.C., and Janicki, B.W. Mitogen-induced blastogenic responses of lymphocytes from marihuana smokers. Science 188:71-72, 1975.

Zimmerman, A.M. and Raj, A.Y. Influence of cannabinoids on somatic cells in vivo. Pharmacology 21:277-287, 1980.

Zimmerman, A.M., Stich, H., and San, R. Nonmutagenic action of cannabinoids in vitro. Pharmacology 16:333-343, 1978.

Zimmerman, A.M., Bruce, W.R., and Zimmerman, S. Effects of cannabinoids on sperm morphology. Pharmacology 18:143-148, 1979.

6

BEHAVIORAL AND PSYCHOSOCIAL EFFECTS
OF MARIJUANA USE

The mind-altering effects of marijuana underlie its widespread and
increasing popularity. Marijuana users who experience effects on
mood, perception, and motivation report that they seek the "high" and
the "mellowing-out." However, under some circumstances many of these
same effects can be considered adverse. Perceptual distortions that
are sought by users pose risks for driving cars or using other
machines. There is reason to be concerned about effects on learning
by students using marijuana in school. Older adults receiving
Δ-9-THC as therapy may be highly intolerant of altered consciousness
and perceived loss of control. Thus, it has become a matter of
practical as well as scientific interest to learn more about the
effects of marijuana on the brain and behavior.

Many psychological and neuropsychological studies have been
conducted to investigate specific effects of marijuana on behavior.
These include studies of intellectual functions, such as memory,
attention, sequential information processing, and decision-making, as
well as perceptual and psychomotor functions. There is a methodological challenge in trying to design experiments that will discriminate
reliably among these functions and determine precisely which is being
affected when a drug produces a particular behavioral outcome. For
example, one's ability to process and respond to environmental stimuli
represents a chain of events. The sequence begins with a sensation
or perception. Drugs can influence the manner, speed, and accuracy
with which this input is received. The information must then be
stored in memory, even if only very briefly, and then retrieved from
memory to be integrated with recalled prior experiences and other
sensory inputs. The response from the subject is the result of the
integration of new and old information. A drug acting at any point
in this chain of events can alter behavioral performance.

Studies of the effects of marijuana on complex behavior must be
carefully interpreted, because there are numerous variables that can
influence the results. First, there is the drug itself. The dose,
type of preparation, route of administration, and speed of administration must be specified. Next, the user--his personality, level of
innate ability, motivation to perform, and especially his previous
experience with marijuana, are powerful influences on test results.
Finally, there is the type of behavioral test and the setting in

which it is performed. Simpler and well-practiced skills are less susceptible to disruption by drug effects than are novel or complex tasks. The studies in the literature vary in their attention to these factors.

Most of these studies have been carried out on male college students who volunteer for marijuana research. Although this age-group (19-25) represents a period of peak use of marijuana, it cannot be assumed that findings from a college population will generalize to other sectors of the youth population. The differing motives of student volunteers seriously confound the interpretation of results in intellectual areas, where it has been established that motivation plays a significant role in determining performance. Some dedicated users want to do well and demonstrate that marijuana has no harmful effect. Others are simply interested in obtaining the drug and enjoying its effects with little interest in the experiment. Additional methodological issues that recur in this body of research include: (a) reliance on self-reports by subjects regarding personal history of frequency and intensity of drug use, (b) occasional reliance on self-reports of drug dose and level of intoxication at the time of the experiment, (c) lack of standardized dosages and methods of administration of Δ-9-THC even when the drug is administered by the investigator, and (d) lack of attention to motives and beliefs of users and nonusers with whom they interact.

A representative sample of studies will be reviewed here, and a summary table of 88 reports of the relationship between marijuana use and behavioral and psychosocial functioning is available from the Institute of Medicine by request.

PERCEPTUAL AND PSYCHOMOTOR FUNCTIONS

Acute Effects

The studies reported here cover the range of commonly used doses* from very low up to 0.250 mg/kg of Δ-9-THC in marijuana cigarettes at a single sitting. These are acute effects--changes that can be seen after a single dose. The effects begin to be seen at about the same dose level at which a "high" is perceived (0.050-0.150 mg/kg Δ-9-THC). Generally the effects are dose-related. In other words, low doses have small effects; higher doses tend to have greater effects.

---

*Doses are reported in milligrams per kilogram (mg/kg) where provided by the authors or as total doses in milligrams with the route of administration.

Coordination

Marijuana has been found to impair motor coordination at doses commonly used in social settings by both naive and chronic users. The functions studied include: hand steadiness (Mayor's Committee on Marihuana, 1944; Clark et al., 1970; Milstein et al., 1975), body sway (Mayor's Committee on Marihuana, 1944; Kiplinger et al., 1971; Evans et al., 1973), and accuracy of execution movements (Rafaelsen et al., 1973; Milstein et al., 1975; Kvalseth, 1977). Studies have also showed a dose-related increase in impairment of postural stability as measured by increased body sway (Kiplinger et al., 1971).

Reaction Time

Reaction time is defined as the time lag between a signal and the response a subject makes to that signal. Most studies examine the time that it takes a subject to respond to a visual or auditory signal. The effects of marijuana on either speed of initial detection of the signal or speed of response have been inconsistent at doses commonly used in social settings ("low to moderate"). The same subjects are impaired at some times, but not at other times (Mayor's Committee on Marihuana, 1944; Clark et al., 1970; Dornbush et al., 1971; Moskowitz et al., 1972, 1974; Borg et al., 1975; Schaefer et al., 1977; Peeke et al., 1976; Stillman et al., 1977). The meaning of this inconsistency is uncertain, but it probably involves an effect on attention mechanisms. When a subject is intoxicated with marijuana, he is probably less likely to attend to the reaction time task. Perhaps it is when he does pay attention to the task that function on this test is not impaired.

Tracking

Tracking is the term used to describe the act of following a moving stimulus. It is an important component of driving and flying skills. Tracking behavior is highly sensitive to the effects of marijuana. Impairment of tracking occurs even at very low doses (4.5 mg by smoking) in naive subjects (Weil et al., 1968). Studies of experienced users have also demonstrated consistent impairment. The tracking impairment has been found to persist for 4 to 8 hours, well beyond the feeling of intoxication ("high") by one laboratory (Moskowitz and Sharma, 1979; Moskowitz et al., 1981). No other studies have measured the effects of marijuana beyond 2 hours. This finding on the long-lasting effects has very important implications, as will be discussed later when the effects of marijuana on driving are reviewed, and, therefore, such studies should be repeated by other investigators.

While reaction time studies (as noted above) showed inconsistent results, tracking behavior is regularly and significantly diminished by marijuana at doses usually used in social settings. Tracking tasks differ from reaction time studies, because the subject must continuously pay attention to the task. Since reaction time tests are intermittent, continuous attention is not required, and this may explain why reaction time studies fail to show consistent marijuana effects.

Sensory and Perceptual Functions

Tests that measure a subject's ability to detect a brief flash of light show significant impairment by low to moderate doses (2-3 mg are examples) of smoked marijuana (Sharma and Moskowitz, 1972, 1973, 1974; Moskowitz et al., 1972, 1974; Casswell and Marks, 1973; Jones and Stone, 1970). Sustained attention is required in signal detection tasks, and the relation between this sustained attention requirement and motivation effects has not been explored. Signal detection tasks are prototypes of perceptual demands found in man-machine interactions. The large reductions in signal detection that occur under the influence of marijuana may suggest a substantial risk for users who are operating machines. Other visual functions, such as visual search, that depend on eye movements are not impaired.

Intellectual and Cognitive Functions

The effects of marijuana on such intellectual and cognitive functions as verbal fluency, short-term memory, learning ability, calculation skills, ability to follow complex directions, and time sense have been investigated and are reported below. However, this area of study has been hampered by the lack of standard measures of functioning in the intellectual and cognitive areas tested. Overall, the investigation of marijuana effects on intellectual and cognitive functioning has not followed a logical progression.

Learning and Memory When studying the effects of drugs on learning, it is difficult to control all of the factors that might influence the results; for example, as noted above, how hard a subject tries to perform can make a big difference even in the presence of a sedating drug. Thus, it is not surprising that early studies of marijuana's effects gave inconsistent results.

More recently, several studies have demonstrated that a single moderate dose of marijuana impairs short-term memory. This effect is especially noticeable in the phases of short-term memory that are heavily dependent on attention, such as information acquisition and storage (Abel, 1970, 1971; Dornbush et al., 1971; Dittrich et al., 1973; Melges et al., 1974; Belmore and Miller, 1980). Examples of the types of impaired tasks would be remembering a sequence of numbers or syllables or memorizing and following a sequence of directions.

Physiological changes have been monitored in some of the same studies in which intellectual impairment has been reported. Miller and Cornett (1978) found that increases in heart rate are produced by marijuana to about the same degree as impairment on intellectual tasks. This linking of a physiological marker with studies of behavioral effects is a useful model for research in this field.

Time Sense   Another intellectual function influenced by marijuana is time sense. Under the influence of moderate doses of the drug, most investigators report that subjects consistently overestimate the amount of time that has elapsed. Thus, under the influence of marijuana, a given event is reported to last longer than it actually does last (Clark et al., 1970; Vachon et al., 1974; Tinklenberg et al., 1976a).

State-Dependent Learning   State-dependent learning refers to a situation in which material that is learned while under the influence of a drug is remembered best in the state of drug intoxication in which it was originally learned. A series of studies were conducted with oral doses of 20 mg (in a subsequent study this dose was calibrated to 0.3 mg/kg) of Δ-9-THC to investigate the extent to which learning and memory are linked to the state of intoxication (Darley et al., 1973a,b, 1974, 1977). This modest dose of marijuana caused learning to take place more slowly than when the subject was drug-free. Once learned, recall of the learning that occurred during intoxication was best when the subject was again under the influence of marijuana. Although state-dependent learning occurs with marijuana, the quality of learning and recall is impaired because the information or problem-solving skills learned in the marijuana-intoxicated state will be reduced or impaired. These investigators believe that the major deficit is in the attention-storage phase of learning.

Oral Communication

Marijuana use in low to moderate doses impairs oral communication, especially clarity of sequential dialogue with other persons (Dornbush et al., 1971; Paul and Carson, 1973; Zeidenberg et al., 1973; Crockett et al., 1976; Miller et al., 1977a-d, 1978a,b, 1979; Pfefferbaum et al., 1977; Miller and Cornett, 1978; Natale et al., 1979; Belmore and Miller, 1980). Marijuana at moderate doses disrupts continuity of speech by impairing short-term memory (6-18 seconds duration) (Belmore and Miller, 1980). Communication while intoxicated is also impaired by the intrusion of irrelevant words and ideas into the stream of communication. When a list of words is learned and then the subjects are asked to recall those words without regard to sequence, words that were never in the original list are inserted during recall more often by subjects given Δ-9-THC than by those who were drug-free (Pfefferbaum et al., 1977; Miller and Cornett, 1978; Miller et al., 1978a,b). Zeidenberg et al. (1973) administered 5 mg Δ-9-THC orally and found that, in a social context, phrases became shorter, speech became slower, and there was greater lag time between the cue to talk and the actual onset of talking. These subjects were also less able to recognize three-letter nonsense syllables to which they had previously been exposed. Further, when experimental subjects were all given the same dose of Δ-9-THC, they reported different subjective levels of intoxication. Those who reported more intoxication showed greater disruption of two-person communication (Paul and Carson, 1973).

Experimental subjects who were asked to tell stories about ambiguous pictures (the Thematic Apperception Test) demonstrated drug impaired organization and integration of stories. The authors reported "a timeless, nonnarrative quality, with greater discontinuity in thought sequence and more frequent inclusion of contradictory ideas" (Roth et al., 1975). When asked to talk for five minutes on any topic, subjects under Δ-9-THC demonstrated decreased variability of language and an increase in personal references, as well as less detailing of items mentioned in the monologue and less critical evaluation of those items (Natale et al., 1979).

Auto Accidents

Simulator Studies

A driving simulator is a laboratory instrument that requires the subject to perform a sample of the behavior required in automobile driving situations. Simulators differ from most of the laboratory studies described above in that complex behavior is required. Although simulators are representative of the multitask character of driving, no one simulator is capable of presenting all aspects of driving simultaneously. The behavior sampled varies across simulators; however, in comparison to car driving situations, the simulator has the advantage of presenting a standard stimulus to all subjects.

Most simulator studies reveal impairment of driving skills following moderately intoxicating doses of marijuana such as 10-15 mg (Crancer et al., 1969; Dott, 1972; Ellingstad et al., 1973; Rafaelsen et al., 1973; Moskowitz et al., 1976; Smiley et al., 1981). These impairments have been reported in simulators that test the perceptual functions as well as those that test motor skills of car control.*

---

*Another type of simulator study examined marijuana's effect on performance in a flying simulator (Janowsky et al., 1976). Subjects smoked marijuana cigarettes with 0.09 mg/kg Δ-9-THC, a dose of Δ-9-THC commonly used in social settings. Significant impairment of short-term memory was noted. Subjects were unable to recall where they were in the execution of a task. On the simulator they tended to forget where they were in a given flight sequence.

Test Courses

Experimental studies of the effects of marijuana on closed course automobile driving performance show that this skill is impaired by marijuana. Car handling skills were reduced, as shown by objective measures (Klonoff, 1974; Hansteen et al., 1976; Attwood, in press). It should be noted that these studies, involving subjects under the influence of marijuana, examined performance in less complex situations than are actually met in real-life driving situations. However, a closed course has the advantages of standard conditions and safety factors. In real-life driving situations, the perceptual and cognitive demands are considerably more complex. The Klonoff (1974) study of driving performance on city streets indicates that smoked marijuana (5-10 mg Δ-9-THC) impairs judgment and concentration in addition to impairing car handling skills.

Accident Surveys

Experimental evidence of impairments caused by marijuana on psychomotor functions, judgment, and motor skills involved in driving has led to research on the relationship of the use of marijuana and automobile accidents. A strongly positive relationship between use of alcohol and increased driving risk has long been established. The techniques used to establish the relationship of alcohol to accidents might appear to offer an excellent paradigm for comparable marijuana-accident research. However, there have been practical reasons why the roadside survey model of using breath samples obtained from accident drivers and comparing those to breath samples of randomly selected drivers who are passing the accident site in the same direction, the same time of day, and same day of the week has not worked for marijuana studies. Whereas there has been 97 percent cooperation for alcohol breath analysis, marijuana determination requires a blood sample, and only a minority of drivers willingly cooperate. Further, marijuana has a quite different body distribution pattern due to its high fat solubility. Delta-9-THC is not only technically quite difficult to detect in samples of body fluid, but it may be active in the nervous system long after it is not detectable in blood. The detrimental effects on driving skills (Moskowitz and Sharma, 1979; Moskowitz et al., 1981) may even persist 4 to 8 hours beyond the time when the user has had subjective feelings of euphoria or sleepiness.

Several reports of accident surveys have recently been published (Teale et al., 1977; Cimbura et al., 1980; McBay and Owens, 1981), but all suffer from the problems discussed above and particularly from the lack of a reasonable comparison group. For example, one study reported that 16 percent of Boston drivers had Δ-9-THC in their blood (Sterling-Smith, 1975). There was no description of the group who declined to give a blood sample but provided breath or urine samples instead. Also, there is no information as to the frequency of finding Δ-9-THC in the blood of those drivers who have not had an accident or otherwise come to police attention. In addition, many users of marijuana also use other drugs so that data are available on only a few subjects who only used marijuana.

In an effort to obtain some reference point for the association of marijuana with accidents as compared with other drugs, Warren et al. (in press) reanalyzed the Cimbura et al. (1980) data. Twelve percent of the fatally injured drivers and pedestrians in that study had been found to have Δ-9-THC in their blood. The presence of other drugs was also determined and a culpability index was developed. A culpability index compares the frequency that a drug is found in drivers assigned responsibility for causing a collision with the frequency in individuals from the same sample who had not caused an accident.

Aspirin was found to have a culpability index of 1.0. That is, it was no more frequent in individuals assigned responsibility for a collision than on those who were not. This is of some significance because it serves as an internal check on the technique, agreeing with the a priori assumption that it would be unlikely for aspirin users to be overrepresented among those responsible for accidents. In contrast, subjects with cannabinoids present in the urine were found to have a culpability index of 1.7, the same culpability level found for the presence of alcohol. This indicates an excess of Δ-9-THC-positive drivers in the category responsible for accidents. The presence of antihistamines produced a culpability index of 1.5, and tranquilizers/antidepressants, 1.8.

Given the difficulties in executing epidemiologic studies where it is so difficult to obtain adequate control groups, it would appear that only tentative conclusions about marijuana's role in accidents can be reached. Supportive evidence that marijuana is a contributing cause of accidents comes from surveys of marijuana users who report they receive a higher-than-average number of tickets for driving violations and are involved in a higher-than-average number of accidents (Johnston, 1980). Nevertheless, the problems described above are yet to be solved. But the culpability index model presents a methodology that may be refined and utilized in future studies.

Alcohol-Marijuana Interactions

Surveys show that marijuana and alcohol are frequently consumed together (Fishburne et al., 1980; Johnston et al., 1980). Thus, it is important to determine what interactions, if any, occur between these two drugs. As both drugs have sedative properties, an additive effect would be expected and has been found in the few systematic investigations of the effects of this combination. One study reported that 0.05 percent blood alcohol level concentration (BAC) increased the impairment produced by 5 mg of smoked Δ-9-THC on tracking behavior (Manno et al., 1971). In a study using two doses of alcohol and two doses of marijuana, even the low dose of alcohol (0.07 percent BAC) and the low dose of Δ-9-THC (1.4 mg) impaired complex tracking in an additive fashion (Hansteen et al., 1976).

Higher doses produced more pronounced decrements. A combination of
Δ-9-THC (0.320 mg/kg) and ethanol (a dose that produces a peak
blood level of less than 0.08 percent BAC) has also produced an
additive effect on the ability to perform on a psychomotor test
(Belgrave et al., 1979). This additive effect would be of concern to
those operating a motor vehicle.

The issue of alcohol-marijuana interactions is an important one,
but currently few data are available. Clearly, more studies of
marijuana's interaction with alcohol and other commonly used drugs
are needed.

Chronic Effects

Animal Studies

Studies of chronic effects are necessary to determine whether a drug
produces changes that persist after administration has stopped. In
view of the theoretical possibility of cumulative or persistent
marijuana effects, it is surprising that only a few laboratories have
conducted experiments involving repeated dosing and testing for
residual effects. Mice injected with 10 mg/kg Δ-9-THC for 20-40
days were found to be persistently impaired in new learning 100 days
after the injections stopped (Radouco-Thomas et al., 1976).
Similarly, rats given 20 mg/kg of Δ-9-THC orally for 180 days had
learning still impaired 2 months after the Δ-9-THC treatment
stopped (Fehr et al., 1976). This was confirmed by the same group in
two subsequent studies (Fehr et al., 1979; Stiglick and Kalant, in
press). Another group of investigators, however, could find no
residual learning effects in monkeys 20 days after stopping
comparable doses of Δ-9-THC (Ferraro and Grilly, 1974).

Human Studies

Clinical reports of memory impairment, lack of concentration,
lethargy, etc., in nonintoxicated chronic users of marijuana have led
to studies in which psychological testing was administered to users
of marijuana and controls. The results of these studies are
inconclusive. Several studies show impaired performance in users as
compared to controls (Agarwal et al., 1975; Soueif, 1976; Wig and
Varma, 1977; Mendhiratta et al., 1978); others found no significant
residual effects in the marijuana users (Bowman and Pihl, 1973; Rubin
and Comitas, 1975; Satz et al., 1976; Ray et al., 1978; Schaeffer et
al., 1981). All of these studies can be criticized on methodological
grounds, and the results have been disputed. This is not surprising,
because it is technically very difficult to obtain a sample of
chronic marijuana users, get them into a truly drug-free condition,
test them, and similarly test an appropriate group of controls.

Several groups of investigators (Dornbush et al., 1972; Frank et
al., 1976; Harshman et al., 1976; Rossi et al., 1977) examined

chronic marijuana users before and after 21-94 days of chronic intoxication in a research hospital setting. None of the investigators found any psychological changes during postdrug testing. However, 2 months of use is a relatively short period of time for a change to be detected, and the subjects had already been using marijuana for at least a year prior to entering each study (Fehr et al., 1976).

The available studies of chronic behavioral effects lead to no clear conclusions. Although some animal studies demonstrated a learning deficit that persisted for months after daily marijuana exposure was discontinued, the human studies have such methodological weaknesses that they cannot be interpreted. A prospective concurrent cohort study and a retrospective case-control study of possible outcomes of and risk factors for use of marijuana could add useful information. (See research recommendations at the end of this chapter.)

CLINICAL SYNDROMES

In this section we will discuss both acute and chronic behavioral changes that have been reported in the clinical literature to be associated with the use of marijuana. An association based on case reports does not imply causality. Studies of appropriate control groups are necessary. In general, acute or immediate clinical effects of drugs can be determined scientifically much more readily than chronic or delayed effects. This is as true for marijuana as it is for alcohol and other drugs. Thus, the acute effects of marijuana are based on more solid evidence than are the reported chronic effects.

Acute Effects

The acute clinical effects of marijuana seem to occur on a continuum from mild dysphoria to acute brain syndrome. In the literature, three different syndromes have been described, although there is blurring of the boundaries in this classification and no general agreement as to diagnostic criteria.

Anxiety/Panic Reaction

A major portion of the evidence for this effect comes from reports by marijuana users themselves. Marijuana's popularity notwithstanding, a surprisingly high proportion of users report reactions that they regard as unpleasant or undesirable. For example, 33 percent of regular users reported that while intoxicated they occasionally experienced such symptoms as acute panic, paranoid reaction, hallucinations, and unpleasant distortions in body image (Tart, 1970; Negrete and Kwan, 1972). Another study reported that 16 percent of regular users reported anxiety, fearfulness, confusion, dependency, or aggressive urges as a "usual occurrence" (Halikas et al., 1971). Similar findings in groups of stable, well-adjusted, moderate users have been found by other investigators (Annis and Smart, 1973; Marcus et al., 1974). First-time users are more likely than are experienced users to report adverse reactions. The frequency of such reactions appears to be higher when the setting for use is not a favorable one; for example, when the user sees the environment as threatening.

These adverse psychological reactions also have been observed in subjects of laboratory experiments with marijuana. Such controlled observations of persons whose immediate prior mental status and whose dosage were known give a basis for concluding that acute adverse psychological reactions can occur under single moderate doses of marijuana. These effects are more likely at higher doses. They usually last no longer than 2 to 4 hours. Acute paranoid reactions under these controlled conditions have been reported (Mendelson and Meyer, 1972; Tassinari et al., 1973; Frank et al., 1976; Melges, 1976). Ingestion, in which titration of dose (dose adjustment as occurs during smoking) is difficult, may be more likely to produce adverse effects than administration by smoking marijuana. However, chronic use and interaction with other psychoactive substances are not required.

As frequently as these adverse reactions are observed and self-reported, medical treatment is rarely sought. For example, a college student health clinic reported only six students per year sought medical treatment for an adverse reaction to marijuana out of a student population of 20,000 (Pillard, 1970). In the general population, a diagnosis of acute cannabis reaction was found in only 10 cases out of 700,000 hospital admissions in the United States (Lundberg et al., 1971). In the U.S. Army, only 18 such cases were treated over a several-year period from a military population of 33,000 (Tennant and Groesbeck, 1972). There are no recent figures showing requests for medical treatment now that the use of marijuana is more intense, widespread, and reaching younger age-groups. However, a unique monitoring of drug causality behavior documenting emergency room encounters conducted by the Drug Enforcement Administration and the National Institute on Drug Abuse (U.S. Department of Health and Human Services, 1979) may in the future provide additional information about the frequency of adverse reactions to use of marijuana.

Dysphoric Reaction

Therapeutic trials have been carried out testing Δ-9-THC as a possible treatment for mood disorders (see Chapter 7). Severe dysphoric reactions characterized by disorientation, catatonialike immobility, acute panic, and heavy sedation have occurred in several patients. The dysphoric symptoms appeared at moderate doses comparable to those used in social settings. They lasted only a few hours and responded to discontinuation of the drug and reassurance of the patients (Kotin et al., 1973; Ablon and Goodwin, 1974).

Similar dysphoric reactions have been reported in cancer patients who were on a therapeutic trial of Δ-9-THC to control the nausea associated with chemotherapy. The symptoms, course, and response to ceasing use of the drug were identical to those described above. Investigators have suggested that the dysphoric response is more likely to occur in older patients not accustomed to drug use for whom the mood-altering effects are unanticipated and unwelcome (Shiling and Stillman, 1980).

Acute Brain Syndrome

Diagnostic criteria for the syndrome now called delirium and previously called acute brain syndrome appear in Diagnostic and Statistical Manual of Mental Disorders, Third Edition, 1980 (DSM III). These include: (a) a clouding of consciousness as manifested by impairment of ability to sustain attention to environmental stimuli, or impairment of ability to sustain goal-directed thinking or goal-directed behavior; (b) a disorder of memory or orientation; (c) perceptual disturbances; and (d) a change in sleep pattern and/or a change in psychomotor activity. The symptoms develop over a short period of time and fluctuate rapidly.

Both the symptom pattern and the course of the acute brain syndrome fit the descriptions of one type of behavior disorder associated with use of marijuana. It has been reported to develop in persons who have a history of prolonged, regular, heavy use of marijuana. It is defined as an "acute" brain syndrome because it comes on during the period of drug use and it gradually disappears after the drug is stopped. The majority of case reports have come from Eastern countries where the cannabis products customarily used have high potency (Spencer, 1970; Chopra and Smith, 1974; Meyer, 1975). It has also been reported in U.S. Army personnel stationed in Viet Nam (Talbott and Teague, 1969) and in Europe (Tennant, 1972), where soldiers had access to very high Δ-9-THC concentrations in cannabis substances. In contrast to the Indian public mental hospital patients who were hospitalized for many weeks, U.S. soldiers recovered in 3 to 11 days and returned to duty. This difference in duration may reflect sociocultural differences in length of in-patient treatment more than a difference in the disorder.

Withdrawal Syndrome

Studies of animals and human subjects given moderate to high doses of marijuana orally or by inhalation several times per day have demonstrated tolerance to many of the effects of marijuana (see Chapter 1). When such use of marijuana is stopped after several days, a withdrawal syndrome occurs. In human subjects, this resembles the typical mild withdrawal symptoms seen after prolonged sedative use (Jones and Benowitz, 1976). Subjects show irritability, agitation, insomnia, and EEG changes (see Chapter 4). These symptoms are self-limiting; they peak at 30 hours and disappear by 90 hours.

There is no clinical evidence that physical dependence plays an important role in persistent use of marijuana. Withdrawal symptoms would not be expected in intermittent users; however, daily round-the-clock users of high-dose marijuana may be expected to show some symptoms of withdrawal soon after stopping regular use.

Chronic Effects

Cannabis Psychosis

Cannabis psychosis refers to a chronic psychotic condition (out of contact with reality) reportedly seen in heavy marijuana users, but extending beyond the period of acute intoxication. Some authors have described a schizophrenialike picture with delusions and hallucinations, and others have stressed the existence of organic mental confusion. Most of the reports have come from observation of hospitalized patients in Asian and African countries (Asuni, 1964; Chopra and Smith, 1974; Thacore and Shukla, 1976). There are no reports in the North American literature. At this time, there is insufficient evidence to say that cannabis psychosis exists as a separate clinical entity (Murphy, 1963; Edwards, 1976).

"Amotivational Syndrome"

Clinicians coined the term "amotivational syndrome" to describe a characteristic set of personality changes seen in some daily users of marijuana (McGlothlin and West, 1968; Smith, 1968). The changes include apathy, loss of ambition, loss of effectiveness, diminished ability to carry out long-term plans, difficulty in concentrating, and a decline in school or work performance. As usually described, these changes are seen in frequent or daily users, and thus they may be considered a form of chronic intoxication. The term "amotivational syndrome" is not an official diagnosis, but there is agreement among many clinicians who treat young people that this constellation of symptoms is common. It may also be seen in nonmarijuana users, and daily use of marijuana is not always associated with loss of motivation.

The evidence presented for the linking of this syndrome with marijuana consists of case reports. For example, Baker and Lucas (1969) described the case of a man whom friends described as previously conscientious, capable, and effective; but after smoking hashish daily for 3 years, he changed into a person for whom use of drugs was a way of life and in whom a serious deterioration of social function was observed. Other reports consist of groups of cases with similar histories (Thurlow, 1971). The symptoms mentioned, in addition to loss of motivation, include falling grades, difficulties in concentration, intermittent confusion, and impaired memory. Some authors report improvement when use of marijuana is stopped (Kolansky and Moore, 1971, 1972).

A variety of other data support such a condition. In a large survey, daily marijuana users were asked about the drug's adverse effects (Johnston et al., 1980). The most common response was "loss of energy" (42 percent). Nearly a third (32 percent) of the daily users thought that marijuana caused them to be less interested in other activities than they had been before, and a third (34 percent) thought that it hurt their school and/or job performance. Another type of evidence comes from comparisons of college students who use marijuana with others who do not. Several such studies (Shean and Fechtmann, 1971; Linn, 1972; Simon, 1974; Finnell and Jones, 1975) found marijuana users had increased levels of psychological disturbance, lower academic performance, and lower performance on scales measuring attitudes toward achievement and purpose in life. But some studies in both the United States and foreign countries have failed to show significant differences between marijuana users and abstainers (Brill and Christie, 1974; Rubin and Comitas, 1975).

Interpretation of the evidence linking marijuana to "amotivational syndrome" is difficult. Such symptoms have been known to occur in the absence of marijuana. Even if there is an association between this syndrome and use of marijuana, that does not prove that marijuana causes the syndrome. Many troubled individuals seek an "escape" into use of drugs; thus, frequent use of marijuana may become one more in a series of counterproductive behaviors for these unhappy people.

The available evidence does not allow a sorting of the various possibilities in the relationship between use of marijuana and the complex of symptoms in the "amotivational syndrome." It appears likely that both self-selection and authentic drug effects contribute to the "motivational" problems seen in some chronic marijuana users (see Chapter 2). Persons who are experiencing loss of motivation, apathy, and the other aforementioned symptoms probably will worsen the situation by taking any sedating drug. They should be warned to avoid frequent use of marijuana, alcohol, and other nonprescribed drugs.

"Flashbacks"

In 1968, Keeler et al. reported four cases of the brief spontaneous recurrence of a mental state similar to that experienced during marijuana intoxication 1 to 21 days after the last drug use. Three of the four subjects complained of hallucinations comparable to flashbacks usually associated with LSD (Horowitz, 1969). Three separate reports of marijuana flashbacks followed (Smith, 1968; Favazza and Domino, 1969; Weil, 1970) and all of these latter subjects had used LSD prior to marijuana. In a survey of 720 servicemen, not a single case of flashback in any subject for whom hashish was the only drug consumed was documented (Tennant and Groesbeck, 1972). But in the same sample, 15 subjects were identified who had LSD flashbacks precipitated by use of marijuana. A larger sample of 2,001 army personnel (Stanton et al., 1976) revealed that use of marijuana had the highest and only statistically significant association with the precipitation of LSD flashbacks among five classes of abused drugs. Clinical studies also have provided evidence that marijuana precipitates a recurrence of the LSD flashbacks experience (Holsten, 1976; Abraham, 1981).

The existence of flashbacks following use of either LSD or marijuana is entirely based on self-reports, because there are no distinctive physical signs or tests, such as EEG changes, to identify this condition. There is no current pharmacological explanation of the phenomenon, and data regarding dose and time parameters do not exist. Still, the reports by users are reasonably consistent. Thus, there is clinical evidence that use of marijuana by those who have previously used LSD increases the likelihood of recurrence of the LSD experience.

Effects on Preexisting Mental Illness

The only evidence available regarding this issue consists of case reports of patients who had recovered and apparently were doing well until they used marijuana. There is no information on the number of mentally ill patients who have used marijuana without complications.

The available data, therefore, do not prove that marijuana worsens mental illness. Still, there are sufficient numbers of uncontrolled clinical reports showing a temporal association between use of marijuana and return of mental symptoms, so that patients should be warned of this possibility.

Patients with a history of schizophrenia may be particularly sensitive to marijuana's effects. Four schizophrenic patients who were otherwise well controlled with medication suffered serious relapse of their schizophrenic symptoms following use of marijuana (Treffert, 1978). Other cases have been reported (Smith and Mehl, 1970; Weil, 1970; Bernhardson and Gunne, 1972). These all were cases in which marijuana was purchased on the street, so the dose and purity were unknown.

Patients with mood disorders have also been reported to show worsening of mental symptoms after use of marijuana. For example, four cases are known in which marijuana apparently precipitated a relapse of psychotic (hypomanic) behavior (Harding and Knight, 1973). Furthermore, depressed patients treated with Δ-9-THC have been observed to show a high incidence of dysphoric reactions (Ablon and Goodwin, 1974).

Effects Sometimes Reported By Users

Mood Changes

There is a general belief that use of marijuana alters mood. This property is one of the desired effects sought by many users. Investigators have described a number of variables that enter into the mood response to marijuana (Jones, 1971). These include dosage, past experience, attitude, expectations, and setting. For example, individuals who used marijuana in isolation tended to be relaxed and slightly drowsy; in contrast, when the user was in a group situation, marijuana was associated with euphoria and lack of sedative effect (Jones, 1971). Further evidence that mood changes are not attributable solely to the pharmacological action of marijuana comes from a study that found that elevation in mood occurred immediately before use of marijuana and immediately after, but that mood was not correlated with other indications of the subjective level of intoxication (Rossi et al., 1978). Instead, mood was correlated significantly with the moods of others, whether or not the other persons were intoxicated.

It appears that preexisting mood can influence the decision to use marijuana. High school students who exhibit symptoms of depression are more likely than are others to begin using marijuana as well as other illicit drugs (Paton et al., 1977). There is some evidence that students use the drug as a self-prescribed remedy for their own mood problems, often reporting that they use marijuana as a means of psychological coping (Johnston et al., 1980; Kaplan, 1980).

A belief that marijuana can be used to alleviate clinical depression is not supported by other studies, including one in which Δ-9-THC was carefully tested as an antidepressant. It was given to depressed patients as an experimental treatment without success (Ablon and Goodwin, 1974) (see Chapter 7).

Interpersonal Behavior

Adolescents and young adults often report that they use marijuana to facilitate interaction in new social situations (Mirin and McKenna, 1975). In a survey of 704 midwestern undergraduate students, most reported that marijuana was a meaningful "tool of social bonding" (Linn, 1971). There seems to be a widespread belief that marijuana smoking has several facilitative effects, including enhanced social effectiveness, closer social bonding, heightened interpersonal sensitivity and empathy, and enhanced sexual pleasure. The subcultural lore on one of these measures of interpersonal behavior-- sexual effects--has not been studied systematically either in surveys or in experimental studies. The effects on sex hormones are controversial (see Chapter 5). Studies in experimental situations have failed to show any enhancement of social interaction and, in fact, some decrements were noted (Galanter et al., 1974; Clopton et al., 1979; Janowsky et al., 1979). Data from natural settings rather than experimental settings are not available.

Effects on Aggression

Because marijuana users have been involved in delinquent behavior, a number of investigators have questioned whether use of marijuana enhances aggressiveness in human beings. There are specific concerns about potential links of use of marijuana to aggression. Both retrospective and experimental studies in human beings have failed to yield evidence that marijuana use leads to increased aggression. Most of these studies suggest quite the contrary effect. Marijuana appears to have a sedative effect, and it may reduce somewhat the intensity of angry feelings and the probability of interpersonal aggressive behavior (McGuire and Megaree, 1974; Tinklenberg, 1974; Salzman et al., 1976; Taylor et al., 1976; Tinklenberg et al., 1976b; Hemphill and Fisher, 1980).

SUMMARY

There is experimental evidence that marijuana seriously impairs psychomotor performance. Strong evidence for impairment has been found in:

* coordination as examined by hand steadiness, body sway, and accuracy of execution of movement;
* tracking performance;
* perceptual tasks;
* vigilance;
* performance on automobile driving and flying simulators; and
* operating automobiles on test roadways.

Less reliable evidence of impairment or reliable evidence of a small degree of impairment was found in reaction time, simple sensory functions, and control of eye movements. Although the effects that marijuana produces on psychomotor functions used in driving are clear, studies linking marijuana to auto accidents are inconclusive. The research is impaired by methodological problems related to the pharmacology of marijuana. One recent study reported that marijuana and alcohol had a similar degree of association with fatal accidents, but more investigation is needed.

Studies also have shown acute effects of marijuana on short-term memory. State-dependent learning also has been shown, in that information or problem-solving skills learned in the intoxicated state will be reduced or impaired in the drug-free state. One laboratory has shown tracking impairment to persist for 4 to 8 hours beyond the feeling of intoxication. Some animal studies demonstrate a learning deficit that persists for months after marijuana exposure has been discontinued, but human studies do not permit secure conclusions.

The acute clinical effects of marijuana are fairly well established, although there is no general agreement as to how to classify them. Anxiety and panic reactions have been reported by users and observed in experimental situations. They are not uncommon, but they rarely require medical attention. When marijuana is used to treat nausea and other conditions, mental effects can occur, which some patients, especially older persons, may regard as unpleasant. These mental effects may require cessation of the treatment.

Marijuana also has been found to produce an acute brain syndrome. This is a more severe mental problem consisting of confusion and loss of contact with reality. It lasts from several hours to several days and appears to be more likely to occur with higher doses.

Chronic effects of any drug are more difficult to assess than are immediate effects. The evidence that marijuana produces a chronic psychosis is not convincing. The possible role of marijuana in causing an amotivational syndrome is a matter of great concern. Apathy, poor school work or work performance, and lack of goals characterize a number of long-term marijuana users. But it has not been possible to determine how much is caused by use of marijuana and how much was antecedent; it seems likely that both factors (drug effect and self-selection) contribute to the motivational problems seen in chronic users of marijuana. Existing studies have produced conflicting results. None of the investigators has looked at effects on the very young daily marijuana user, who is regarded as potentially at high risk for damaging effects because of physiological and psychological immaturity.

There is clinical evidence that marijuana use by former LSD users may precipitate a recurrence of LSD-type hallucinations known as a "flashback." Other clinical evidence raises the possibility that marijuana use can worsen preexisting mental illness.

RECOMMENDATIONS FOR RESEARCH

The committee recommends the following types of studies.

* Systematic research on acute behavioral and psychosocial effects of marijuana should be extended to other age groups. There are virtually no data on prepubertal children, young adolescents, older adults, and aging persons.
* Studies of effects of daily use of marijuana on school children are greatly needed. These effects should include the learning of new material, physical, psychological, and social development, acquisition of coping skills, and tools of daily living.
* Systematic studies of long-term effects of marijuana are increasingly possible now that longitudinal studies have identified representative panels of persons known to be chronic heavy users. These studies should cover interactive effects of marijuana and other drugs on behavioral and psychosocial responses, especially interactions of alcohol and marijuana because of their frequency of associated use.
* Dosage effects should be restudied, taking into account the higher potency cannabis that is in current use. Further study is needed of the timing and depth of inhalation of cigarettes with standard doses of marijuana. More animal studies at varying doses are needed. In view of the long-term retention of marijuana in body tissues, further study is needed to see whether or not chronic users may have impairments of function even in the absence of an acute dose

of marijuana. The factors that influence the persistence of effects following an acute dose are not understood.

　　• The correlation of changes in a physiological marker, such as increased heart rate, with observations of behavioral effects should be encouraged.

　　• Many of these recommendations, along with those of other chapters, could be consolidated and carried out as part of a study that is both a prospective cohort study and a retrospective case-control study of possible outcomes and risk factors with marijuana use.

　　• A cohort of drug-naive junior high school students could be assembled and followed over time to see which students become marijuana users and which remain nonusers. Students would be subjected to physical and psychosocial testing at predetermined time intervals. The two groups would be evaluated in terms of the incidence of specific outcomes and the relative risks associated with these outcomes after appropriate follow-up periods.

In order to identify risk factors for marijuana use, individuals who become marijuana users would be compared to individuals who remain nonusers using a case-control methodology. By combining these two epidemiologic research strategies, the etiology and effects of marijuana use may be studied.

REFERENCES

Abel, E.L. Marijuana and memory. Nature 227:1151-1152, 1970.

Abel, E.L. Effects of marihuana on the solution of anagrams, memory, and appetite. Nature 231:260-261, 1971.

Ablon, S.L. and Goodwin, F.K. High frequency of dysphoric reactions to tetrahydrocannabinol among depressed patients. Am. J. Psychiatry 131:448-453, 1974.

Abraham, H.D. Visual disturbances in population of LSD users, Paper presented at the 134th Annual Meeting of the American Psychiatric Association, New Orleans, May 14, 1981.

Agarwal, A.K., Sethi, B.B., and Gupta, S.C. Physical and cognitive effects of chronic bhang (cannabis) intake. Indian J. Psychiatry 17:1-7, 1975.

Annis, H.M. and Smart, R.G. Adverse reactions and recurrences for marijuana use. Br. J. Addict. 68:315-319, 1973.

Asuni, T. Socio-psychiatric problems of cannabis in Nigeria. Bull. Narcotics 16:17-28, 1964.

Attwood, D.A. Cannabis, alcohol and driving: Effects on selected closed-course tasks. In Proceedings of the 8th International Conference on Alcohol, Drugs and Traffic Safety, June 15-19, 1980, Stockholm, Sweden (in press).

Baker, A.A. and Lucas, E.G. Some hospital admissions associated with cannabis. Lancet 1:148, 1969.

Belgrave, B.E., Bird, K.D., Chesher, G.B., et al. The effects of (-)trans-Δ-9-tetrahydrocannabinol, alone and in combination with ethanol, on human performance. <u>Psychopharmacology</u> 62:53-60, 1979.

Belmore, S.M. and Miller, L.L. Levels of processing and acute effects of marijuana on memory. <u>Pharmacol. Biochem. Behav.</u> 13:199-203, 1980.

Bernhardson, G. and Gunne, L.M. Forty-six cases of psychosis in cannabis abusers. <u>Int. J. Addict.</u> 7:9-16, 1972.

Borg, J., Gershon, S., and Alpert, M. Dose effects of smoked marihuana on human cognitive and motor functions. <u>Psychopharmacologia</u> 42:211-218, 1975.

Bowman, M. and Pihl, R.O. Cannabis: Psychological effects of chronic heavy use. A controlled study of intellectual functioning in chronic users of high potency cannabis. <u>Psychopharmacologia</u> 29:159-170, 1973.

Brill, N.Q. and Christie, R.L. Marihuana use and psychosocial adaptation. <u>Arch. Gen. Psychiatry</u> 31:713-719, 1974.

Casswell, S. and Marks, D. Cannabis induced impairment of performance of a divided attention task. <u>Nature</u> 241:60-61, 1973.

Chopra, G.S. and Smith, J.W. Psychotic reactions following cannabis use in East Indians. <u>Arch. Gen. Psychiatry</u> 30:24-27, 1974.

Cimbura, G., Warren, R.A., Bennett, R.C., et al. <u>Drugs Detected in Fatally Injured Drivers and Pedestrians in the Province of Ontario</u> Ottawa, Ontario: Traffic Injury Research Foundation of Canada, 1980.

Clark, L.D., Hughes, R., and Nakashima, E.N. Behavioral effects of marijuana: Experimental studies. <u>Arch. Gen. Psychiatry</u> 23:193-198, 1970.

Clopton, P.L., Janowsky, D.S., Clopton, J.M., et al. Marijuana and the perception of affect. <u>Psychopharmacology</u> 61:203-206, 1979.

Crancer, A., Dille, J.M., Delay, J.C., et al. Comparison of the effects of marihuana and alcohol on simulated driving performance. <u>Science</u> 164:851-854, 1969.

Crockett, D., Klonoff, H., and Clark, C. The effects of marijuana on verbalization and thought processes. <u>J. Pers. Assess.</u> 40:582-587, 1976.

Darley, C.F., Tinklenberg, J.R., Hollister, L.E., and Atkinson, R.C. Marihuana and retrieval from short-term memory. <u>Psychopharmacologia</u> 29:231-238, 1973a.

Darley, C.F., Tinklenberg, J.R., Roth, W.T., et al. Influence of marihuana on storage and retrieval processes in memory. <u>Mem. Cognit.</u> 1:196-200, 1973b.

Darley, C.F., Tinklenberg, J.R., Roth, W.T., and Atkinson, R.C. The nature of storage deficits and state-dependent retrieval under marihuana. <u>Psychopharmacologia</u> 37:139-149, 1974.

Darley, C.F., Tinklenberg, J.R., Roth, W.T., et al. Marijuana effects on long-term memory assessment and retrieval. <u>Psychopharmacology</u> 52:239-241, 1977.

<u>Diagnostic and Statistical Manual of Mental Disorder</u>, Third Edition (DSM III). Washington, D.C.: American Psychiatric Association, 1980.

Dott, A.B. Effect of Marijuana on Risk Acceptance in a Simulated Passing Task. DHEW Publication No. (HSM) 72-10010. Washington, D.C.: U.S. Government Printing Office, 1972.

Dittrich, A., Battig, K., and Zeppelin, I.V. Effects of (-)-Δ^9-tetrahydrocannabinol (Δ^9-THC) on memory, attention and subjective state. Psychopharmacologia 33:369-376, 1973.

Dornbush, R.L., Fink, M., and Freedman, A.M. Marijuana, memory, and perception. Am. J. Psychiatry 128:194-197, 1971.

Dornbush, R.L., Clare, G., Zaks, G., et al. 21-Day administration of marijuana in male volunteers, pp. 115-128. In Lewis, M.F. (ed.) Current Research in Marijuana. New York: Academic Press, 1972.

Edwards, G. Cannabis and the psychiatric position, pp. 321-340. In Graham, J.D.P. (ed.) Cannabis and Health. New York: Academic Press, 1976.

Ellingstad, V.S., McFarling, L.H., and Struckman, D.L. Alcohol, Marijuana and Risk Taking. Contract No. DOT-HS-191-2-301. University of South Dakota, Vermillion, 1973.

Evans, M.A., Martz, R., Brown, D.J., et al. Impairment of performance with low doses of marihuana. Clin. Pharmacol. Ther. 14:936-940, 1973.

Favazza, A.R. and Domino, E.F. Recurrent LSD experience (flashbacks) triggered by marihuana. Univ. Mich. Med. Cent. J. 35:214-216, 1969.

Fehr, K.A., Kalant, H., Leblanc, A.E., and Knox, G.V. Permanent learning impairment after chronic heavy exposure to cannabis or ethanol in the rat, pp. 495-505. In Nahas, G.G. (ed.) Marihuana: Chemistry, Biochemistry, and Cellular Effects. New York: Springer-Verlag, 1976.

Fehr, K.O., Kalant, H., and Knox, G.V. Residual effects of high-dose cannabis treatment on learning muricidal behavior and neurophysiological correlates in rats, pp. 681-691. In Nahas, G.G. and Paton, W.D.M. (eds.) Marihuana: Biological Effects. Analysis, Metabolism, Cellular Responses Reproduction and Brain. Oxford: Pergamon Press, 1979.

Ferraro, D.P. and Grilly, D.M. Effects of chronic exposure to Δ-9-tetrahydrocannabinol on delayed matching-to-sample in chimpanzees. Psychopharmacologia 37:127-138, 1974.

Finnell, W.S. and Jones, J.D. Marijuana, alcohol and academic performance. J. Drug Educ. 5:13-21, 1975.

Fishburne, P.M., Abelson, H.I., and Cisin, I. National Survey on Drug Abuse: Main Findings: 1979. DHHS Publication No. (ADM) 80-976. Washington, D.C.: U.S. Government Printing Office, 1980.

Frank, I.M., Lessin, P.J., Tyrrell, E.D., et al. Acute and cumulative effects of marihuana smoking in hospitalized subjects: A 36-day study, pp. 673-679. In Braude, M.C. and Szara, S. (eds.) Pharmacology of Marihuana. New York: Raven Press, 1976.

Galanter, M., Stillman, R., Wyatt, R.J., et al. Marihuana and social behavior. A controlled study. Arch. Gen. Psychiatry 30:518-521, 1974.

Halikas, J.A., Goodwin, D.W., and Guze, S.B. Marijuana effects: A survey of regular users. JAMA 217:692-694, 1971.

Hansteen, R.W., Miller, R.D., Lonero, L., et al. Effects of cannabis and alcohol on automobile driving and psychomotor tracking. Ann. N.Y. Acad. Sci. 282:240-256, 1976.

Harding, T. and Knight, F. Marihuana-modified mania. Arch. Gen. Psychiatry 29:635-637, 1973.

Harshman, R.A., Crawford, H.J., and Hecht, E. Marihuana, cognitive style, and lateralized hemispheric functions, pp. 205-254. In Cohen, S. and Stillman, R.C. (eds.) The Therapeutic Potential of Marihuana. New York: Plenum Medical Book, 1976.

Hemphill, R.E. and Fisher, W. Drugs, alcohol and violence in 604 male offenders referred for inpatient psychiatric assessment. S. Afr. Med. J. 57:243-247, 1980.

Holsten, F. Flashbacks: A personal follow-up. Arch. Psychiat. Nervenkr. 222:293-304, 1976.

Horowitz, M.J. Flashbacks: Recurrent intrusive images after the use of LSD. Am. J. Psychiatry 126:565-569, 1969.

Janowsky, D.S., Meachom, M.P., Blaine, J.D., et al. Marijuana effects on simulated flying ability. Am. J. Psychiatry 133:384-388, 1976.

Janowsky, D.S., Clopton, P.L., Leichner, P.O., et al. Interpersonal effects of marijuana. Arch. Gen. Psychiatry 36:781-785, 1979.

Johnston, L.D. The daily marijuana user. Paper presented at the meeting of the National Alcohol and Drug Coalition, Washington, D.C., September 18, 1980.

Johnston, L.D., Bachman, J.G., and O'Malley, P.M. Highlights from Student Drug Use in America, 1975-1980. DHHS Publication No. (ADM)81-1066. Washington, D.C.: U.S. Government Printing Office, 1980.

Jones, R.T. Marihuana-induced "high": Influence of expectation, setting and previous drug experience. Pharmacol. Rev. 23:359-369, 1971.

Jones, R.T. and Benowitz, N. The 30-day trip--Clinical studies of cannabis tolerance and dependence, pp. 627-642. In Braude, M.C. and Szara, S. (eds.) Pharmacology of Marihuana. New York: Raven Press, 1976.

Jones, R.T. and Stone, G.C. Psychological studies of marijuana and alcohol in man. Psychopharmacologia 18:108-117, 1970.

Kaplan, H.B. Deviant Behavior in Defense of Self. New York: Academic Press, 1980.

Keeler, M.H., Reifler, C.B., and Liptzin, M.B. Spontaneous recurrence of marihuana effect. Amer. J. Psychiatry 125:384-386, 1968.

Kiplinger, G.F., Manno, J.E., Rodda, B.E., and Forney, R.D. Dose-response analysis of the effects of tetrahydrocannabinol in man. Clin. Pharmacol. Ther. 12:650-657, 1971.

Klonoff, H. Effects of marijuana on driving in a restricted area and on city streets: Driving performance and physiological changes, pp. 359-379. In Miller, L.L. (ed.) Marijuana: Effects on Human Behavior. New York: Academic Press, 1974.

Kolansky, H. and Moore, W.T. Effects of markhuana on adolescents and young adults. _JAMA_ 216:486-492, 1971.

Kolansky, H. and Moore, W.T. Toxic effects of chronic marihuana use. _JAMA_ 222:35-41, 1972.

Kotin, J., Post, R.M., and Goodwin, F.K. Delta-9-tetrahydrocannabinol in depressed patients. _Arch. Gen. Psychiatry_ 28:345-348, 1973.

Kvalseth, T.O. Effects of marijuana on human reaction time and motor control. _Percept. Mot. Skills_ 45:935-939, 1977.

Linn, L.S. Social identification and the use of marijuana. _Int. J. Addict._ 6:79-107, 1971.

Linn, L.S. Psychopathology and experience with marijuana. _Br. J. Addict._ 67:55-64, 1972.

Lundberg, G.D., Adelson, J., and Prosnitz, E.H. Marijuana-induced hospitalization. _JAMA_ 215:121, 1971.

McBay, A.J. and Owens, S.M. Marihuana and driving, pp. 257-263. In Harris, L.S. (ed.) _Problems of Drug Dependence, 1980._ NIDA Research Monograph No.34. DHHS Publication No. (ADM) 81-1058. Washington, D.C.: U.S. Government Printing Office, 1981.

McGlothlin, W.H. and West, L.J. The marijuana problem: An overview. _Am. J. Psychiatry_ 125:370-378, 1968.

McGuire, J.S. and Megaree, E.I. Personality correlates of marijuana use among youthful offenders. _J. Consult. Clin. Psychol._ 42:124-133, 1974.

Manno, J.E., Kiplinger, G.F., Scholz, N., et al. The influence of alcohol and marihuana on motor and mental performance. _Clin. Pharmacol. Ther._ 12:202-211, 1971.

Marcus, A.M., Klonoff, H., and Low, M. Psychiatric status of the marihuana user. _Can. Psychiatr. Assoc. J._ 19:31-39, 1974.

Mayor's Committee on Marihuana. _The Marihuana Problem in the City of New York. Sociological, Medical, Psychological and Pharmacological Studies._ Lancaster, Pa.: Jaques Cattell Press, 1944.

Melges, F.T., Tinklenberg, J.R., Deardorff, C.M., et al. Temporal disorganization and delusional-like ideation. _Arch. Gen. Psychiatry_ 30:855-861, 1974.

Melges, F.T. Tracking difficulties and paranoid ideation during hashish and alcohol intoxication. _Am. J. Psychiatry_ 133:1024-1028, 1976.

Mendelson, J. and Meyer, R. Behavioral and biological concomitants of chronic marihuana smoking by heavy and casual users. _Technical Papers of the First Report of the National Committee on Marihuana and Drug Abuse_, pp. 68-246. Washington, D.C.: U.S. Government Printing Office, 1972.

Mendhiratta, S.S., Wig, N.N., and Varma, S.K. Some psychological correlates of long-term heavy cannabis users. _Br. J. Psychiatry_ 132:482-486, 1978.

Meyer, R.E. Psychiatric consequences of marijuana use: The state of the evidence, pp. 133-152. In Tinklenberg, J.R. (ed.) _Marijuana and Health Hazards: Methodological Issues in Current Research._ New York: Academic Press, Inc., 1975.

Miller, L.L., Cornett, T.L., Brightwell, D.R., et al. Marijuana: Effects on storage and retrieval of prose material. Psychopharmacology 51:311-316, 1977a.

Miller, L., Cornett, T., Drew, W., et al. Marijuana: Dose-response effects on pulse rate, subjective estimates of potency, pleasantness, and recognition memory. Pharmacology 15:268-275, 1977b.

Miller, L.L., McFarland, D.J., Cornett, T.L., et al. Marijuana: Effects on free recall and subjective organization of pictures and words. Psychopharmacology 55:257-262, 1977c.

Miller, L.L., McFarland, D., Cornett, T.L., and Brightwell, D. Marijuana and memory impairment: Effect on free recall and recognition memory. Pharmacol. Biochem. Behav. 7:99-103, 1977d.

Miller, L.L. and Cornett, T.L. Marijuana: Dose effects on pulse rate, subjective estimates of intoxication, free recall and recognition memory. Pharmacol. Biochem. Behav. 9:573-577, 1978.

Miller, L., Cornett, T.L., and McFarland, D. Marijuana: An analysis of storage and retrieval deficits in memory with the technique of restricted reminding. Pharmacol. Biochem. Behav. 8:327-332, 1978a.

Miller, L., Cornett, T.L., and Nallan, G. Marijuana: Effect on nonverbal free recall as a function of field dependence. Psychopharmacology 58:297-301, 1978b.

Miller, L.L., Cornett, T.L., and Wikler, A. Marijuana: Effects on pulse rate, subjective estimates of intoxication and multiple measures of memory. Life Sci. 25:1325-1330, 1979.

Milstein, S.L., MacCannell, K., Karr, G., and Clark, S. Marijuana-produced impairments in coordination. J. Nerv. Ment. Dis. 161:26-31, 1975.

Mirin, S.M. and McKenna, G.J. Combat zone adjustment: The role of marihuana use. Milit. Med. 140:482-485, 1975.

Moskowitz, H., Sharma, S., and McGlothlin, W. Effect of marihuana upon peripheral vision as a function of the information processing demands in central vision. Percept. Mot. Skills 35:875-882, 1972.

Moskowitz, H., Shea, R., and Burns, M. Effect of marihuana on the psychological refractory period. Percept. Mot. Skills 38:959-962, 1974.

Moskowitz, H., Ziedman, K., and Sharma, S. Visual search behavior while viewing driving scenes under the influence of alcohol and marihuana. Hum. Factors 18:417-432, 1976.

Moskowitz, H. and Sharma, S. The effects of marihuana on skills performance. Report to the National Institute on Drug Abuse, Contract No. 271-76-3316, Southern California Research Institute, Los Angeles, Calif., 1979.

Moskowitz, H., Sharma, S., and Ziedman, K. Duration of skills performance impairment under marijuana. American Association for Automotive Medicine Proceedings, October 1-3, 1981, pp. 87-96. San Francisco, Calif..

Murphy, H.B.M. The cannabis habit: A review of recent psychiatric literature. Bull. Narc. 15:15-23, 1963.

Natale, M., Zeidenberg, P., and Jaffe, J. Delta-9-tetrahydrocannibinol: Acute effects on defensive and primary-process language. Int. J. Addict. 14:877-889, 1979.

Negrete, J.C. and Kwan, M.W. Relative value of various etiological factors in short lasting, adverse psychological reactions to cannabis smoking. Int. Pharmacopsychiat. 7:249-259, 1972.

Paton, S., Kessler, R., and Kandel, D. Depressive mood and adolescent illicit drug use: A longitudinal analysis. J. Genet. Psychol. 131:267-289, 1977.

Paul, M.I. and Carson, I.M. Marihuana and communication. Lancet 2:270-271, 1973.

Peeke, S.C., Jones, R.T., and Stone, G.C. Effects of practice on marijuana-induced changes in reaction time. Psychopharmacology 48:159-163, 1976.

Pfefferbaum, A., Darley, C.F., Tinklenberg, J.R., et al. Marijuana and memory intrusions. J. Nerv. Ment. Dis. 165:381-386, 1977.

Pillard, R.C. Marijuana. N. Engl. J. Med. 283:294-303, 1970.

Radouco-Thomas, S., Magnan, F., Grove, R.N., et al. Effect of chronic administration of Δ^1-tetrahydrocannabinol on learning and memory in develping mice, pp. 487-498. In Braude, M.C. and Szara, S. (eds.) Pharmacology of Marihuana. New York: Raven Press, 1976.

Rafaelsen, L., Christrup, H., Bech, P., and Rafaelsen, O.J. Effects of cannabis and alcohol on psychological tests. Nature 242:117-118, 1973.

Ray, R., Prabhu, G.G., Mohan, D., et al. The association between chronic cannabis use and cognitive functions. Drug Alcohol Dependence 3:365-368, 1978.

Rossi, A.M., Kuehnle, J.C., and Mendelson, J.H. Effects of marihuana on reaction time and short-term memory in human volunteers. Pharmacol. Biochem. Behav. 6:73-77, 1977.

Rossi, A.M., Kuehnle, J.C., and Mendelson, J.H. Marihuana and mood in human volunteers. Pharmacol. Biochem. Behav. 8:447-453, 1978.

Roth, W.T., Rosenbloom, M.J., Darley, C.F., et al. Marihuana effects on TAT form and content. Psychopharmacologia 43:261-266, 1975.

Rubin, V. and Comitas, L. Ganja in Jamaica: A Medical Anthropological Study of Chronic Marijuana Use. The Hague: Mouton and Co., 1975.

Salzman, C., Van Der Kolk, B.A., and Shader, R.I. Marijuana and hostility in a small-group setting. Am. J. Psychiatry 133:1029-1033, 1976.

Satz, P., Fletcher, J.M., and Sutker, L.S. Neuropsychologic, intellectual, and personality correlates of chronic marijuana use in native Costa Ricans. Ann. N.Y. Acad. Sci. 282:266-306, 1976.

Schaefer, C.F., Gunn, C.G., and Dubowski, K.M. Dose-related heart-rate, perceptual, and decisional changes in man following marihuana smoking. Percept. Mot. Skills 44:3-16, 1977.

Schaeffer, J., Andrysiak, T., and Ungerleides, J.T. Cogention and long-term use of gauja (cannabis). Science 213:465-466, 1981.

Sharma, S. and Moskowitz, H. Effect of marihuana on the visual autokinetic phenomenon. Percept. Mot. Skills 35:891-894, 1972.

Sharma, S. and Moskowitz, H. Marihuana Dose Study of Vigilance Performance, <u>Proceedings,</u> 81st Annual Conference, American Psychological Association, pp. 1035-1036, 1973.

Sharma, S. and Moskowitz, H. Effects of two levels of attention demand on vigilance performance under marihuana. <u>Percept. Mot. Skills</u> 38:967-970, 1974.

Shean, G.D. and Fechtmann, F. Purpose in life scores of student marihuana users. <u>J. Clin. Psychol.</u> 27:112-113, 1971.

Shiling, D.J. and Stillman, R.C. (moderators). Psychological effects of THC in cancer. Paper session at the 133rd American Psychiatric Association annual meeting, San Francisco, California, May 6, 1980.

Simon, W.E. Psychological needs, academic achievement and marijuana consumption. <u>J. Clin. Psychol.</u> 30:496-498, 1974.

Smiley, A., Ziedman, K., and Moskowitz, H. Pharmacokinetics of drug effects on driving performance: driving simulator tests of marihuana alone and in combination with alcohol. Report to the National Institute on Drug Abuse, Contract No. 271-76-3316, 1981.

Smith, D.E. The acute and chronic toxicity of marijuana. <u>J. Psychadelic Drugs</u> 2:37-47, 1968.

Smith, D.E. and Mehl, C. An analysis of marijuana toxicity. <u>Clin. Toxicol.</u> 3:101-115, 1970.

Soueif, M.I. Some determinants of psychological deficits associated with chronic cannabis consumption. <u>Bull. Narc.</u> 28:25-42, 1976.

Spencer, D.J. Cannabis-induced psychosis. <u>Br. J. Addict.</u> 65:369-372, 1970.

Stanton, M.D., Mintz, J., and Franklin, R.M. Drug flashbacks. II. Some additional findings. <u>Int. J. Addict.</u> 11:53-69, 1976.

Sterling-Smith, R.S. Alcohol, marihuana and other drug patterns among pperators involved in fatal motor vehicle accidents, pp. 93-105. In Israelstam, S. and Lambert, S., eds. <u>Alcohol, Drugs and Traffic Safety</u>. Toronto: Addictive Research Foundation of Ontario, 1975.

Stiglick, A. and Kalant, H. Learning impairment in the radial-arm maze following prolonged cannabis treatment in rats. <u>Psychopharmacology</u> (in press).

Stillman, R.C., Wolkowitz, O., Weingartner, H., et al. Marijuana: Differential effects on right and left hemisphere functions in man. <u>Life Sci.</u> 21:1793-1800, 1977.

Talbott, J.A. and Teague, J.W. Marihuana psychosis: Acute toxic psychosis associated with the use of cannabis derivatives. <u>JAMA</u> 210:299-302, 1969.

Tart, C.T. Marijuana intoxication: Common experiences. <u>Nature</u> 226:701-704, 1970.

Tassinari, C.A., Ambrosetto, G., and Gastaut, H. Effects of marijuana and delta-9-THC at high doses in man. <u>Electroencephalogr. Clin. Neurophysiol.</u> 34:760, 1973.

Taylor, S.P., Vardaris, R.M., Rawtich, A.B., et al. The effects of alcohol and delta-9-tetrahydrocannabinol on human physical aggression. <u>Aggressive Behav.</u> 2:153-161, 1976.

138

Teale, J.D., Clough, J.M., King, L.J., et al. The incidence of cannabinoids in fatally injured drivers: An investigation by radioimmunoassay and high pressure liquid chromatography. J. Forens. Sci. Soc. 17:177-183, 1977.

Tennant, F.S. Drug abuse in the U.S. Army, Europe. JAMA 221:1146-1149, 1972.

Tennant, F.S. and Groesbeck, C.J. Psychiatric effects of hashish. Arch. Gen. Psychiatry 27:133-136, 1972.

Thacore, V.R. and Shukla, S.R.P. Cannabis psychosis and paranoid schizophrenia. Arch. Gen. Psychiatry 33:383-386, 1976.

Thurlow, H.J. On drive state and cannabis: A clinical observation. Can. Psychiatr. Assoc. J. 16:181-182, 1971.

Tinklenberg, J.R. Marijuana and human aggression, pp. 339-357. In Miller, L.L. (ed.) Marijuana: Effects on Human Behavior. New York: Academic Press, 1974.

Tinklenberg, J.R., Roth, W.T., and Kopell, B.S. Marijuana and ethanol: Differential efects on time perception, heart rate, and subjective response. Psychopharmacology 49:275-279, 1976a.

Tinklenberg, J.R., Roth, W.T., Kopell, B.S., and Murphy, P. Cannabis and alcohol effects on assaultiveness in adolescent delinquents. Ann. N.Y. Acad. Sci. 282:85-94, 1976b.

Treffert, D.A. Marijuana use in schizophrenia: A clear hazard. Am. J. Psychiatry 135:1213-1215, 1978.

U.S. Department of Health and Human Services, National Institute on Drug Abuse. Project DAWN. Annual Report--1979. Washington, D.C.: U.S. Government Printing Office, 1979.

Vachon, L., Sulkowski, A., and Rich, E. Marihuana effects on learning, attention and time estimation. Psychopharmacologia 39:1-11, 1974.

Warren, R., Simpson, H., Cimbura, G., et al. Drug Involvement in traffic fatalities in the province of Ontario. Proceedings of the 24th Conference of the American Association for Automotive Medicine (in press).

Weil, A.T., Zinberg, N.E., and Nelsen, J.M. Clinical and psychological effects of marihuana in man. Science 162:1234-1242, 1968.

Weil, A.T. Adverse reactions to marihuana, classification and suggested treatment. N. Engl. J. Med. 282:997-1000, 1970.

Wig, N.N. and Varma, V.K. Patterns of long-term heavy cannabis use in North India and its effects on cognitive functions: A preliminary report. Drug and Alcohol Dependence 2:211-219, 1977.

Zeidenberg, P., Clark, W.C., Jaffe, J., et al. Effect of oral administration of delta-9-tetrahydrocannabinol on memory, speech, and perception of thermal stimulation: Results with four normal human volunteer subjects. Preliminary report. Compr. Psychiatry 14:549-556, 1973.

7

THERAPEUTIC POTENTIAL AND MEDICAL USES OF MARIJUANA

There has been growing interest in the possibility that cannabis and its derivatives will be valuable for the treatment of several medical and psychiatric conditions. The 97th Congress, for example, introduced a bill (H.R. 4498) "to provide for the therapeutic use of marijuana in situations involving life-threatening or sense-threatening illness and to provide adequate supplies of marijuana for such use."

Most of the putative therapeutic effects of cannabis are believed to be mediated by the central nervous system. These include effects on appetite, nausea and vomiting, epilepsy, muscle spasticity, anxiety, depression, pain, and on glaucoma, asthma, and the symptoms of withdrawal from alcohol and narcotics. The literature on these and other therapeutic actions believed mediated by the central nervous system will be reviewed in this chapter.

In general, the committee finds that cannabis shows promise in some of these areas, although the dose necessary to produce the desired therapeutic effect is often close to one that produces an unacceptable frequency of toxic (undesirable) side-effects. What is perhaps more encouraging than the therapeutic effects observed thus far is that cannabis seems to exert its beneficial effects through mechanisms that differ from those of other available drugs. This raises the possibility that some patients who would not be helped by conventional therapies could be treated effectively with cannabis. A second possibility is that cannabis could be combined with other drugs to achieve a therapeutic goal, but with each drug being used at a lower dose than would be required if either were used alone. As a result, fewer side-effects would be expected to occur. It may be possible to reduce side-effects by synthesizing related molecules that could have a more favorable ratio of desired to undesired actions; this line of investigation should have high priority, because such synthetic derivatives may ultimately have widespread therapeutic use.

GLAUCOMA

Glaucoma is the leading cause of blindness in the United States. The term is used to describe a group of ocular diseases characterized by an increase in intraocular pressure, which damages the optic nerve and leads eventually to loss of vision. The disease affects over two million Americans of age 35 or older. Although there is increasing risk of glaucoma with increasing age, there are forms that develop in infancy. The National Society to Prevent Blindness (1980) also estimates that 300,000 new cases are diagnosed each year.

Treatment of glaucoma depends on the type and cause. It may be pharmacological or surgical. Surgery is useful treatment in relatively few cases; there is a high incidence of failure and serious complications may occur. Available antiglaucoma drugs are effective in regulating intraocular pressure in many patients, and are the mainstay of treatment in the most common form of glaucoma, but there are some adverse side-effects. Some patients are refractory to present forms of treatment and become blind as the disease progresses; for them, there is a particularly urgent need to find effective drugs.

Cannabis (the crude drug), Δ-9-THC (the pure compound), and some other cannabinoid derivatives lower intraocular pressure when administered by various routes, such as inhalation, oral, or intravenous. However, adverse side-effects of cannabis and Δ-9-THC also have been reported. Most patients with glaucoma are elderly, and have a reduced tolerance for many of these side-effects. Even without the adverse side effects, smoking, oral, and intravenous routes of administration are not suitable for the long term. For example, to give adequate control for intraocular pressure, four marijuana cigarettes per day of 2 percent Δ-9-THC would be necessary; this amount is considered heavy usage and could pose a serious health problem in long-term use. Therefore, topical application would be the most salutary route of administration for the patient who needs continuous treatment.

Human Studies

Interest in using cannabis for the treatment of glaucoma was first stimulated by the observation of Hepler et al. (1971, 1972) that intraocular pressure decreased when healthy human subjects smoked cannabis (0.9 percent and 1.5 percent Δ-9-THC content) using an ice-cooled water pipe. (See Green, 1979, for an extensive literature review.)

A study of the acute ocular effects of cannabis in 429 subjects showed there was a dose-related and statistically significant reduction of intraocular pressure following the smoking or ingestion of cannabis containing 1, 2, or 4 percent Δ-9-THC (Hepler et al., 1976a). The amount of pressure decrease was in the range of 30 percent for the cannabis that contained 2 percent Δ-9-THC. Nineteen hospitalized subjects who smoked cannabis of 1 or 2 percent

Δ-9-THC content were observed for 35 days and another 29 subjects were observed as in-patients for a total of 94 days. There was a consistent drop in intraocular pressure in those smoking the 2 percent cannabis and the reduction appeared to last 4 to 5 hours (Hepler et al., 1976a). The authors noted that there did not seem to be much of a cumulative effect on size of pupils or upon intraocular pressure response. Studies by other investigators have confirmed this effect of cannabis and Δ-9-THC in causing reduction of intraocular pressure in humans (Shapiro, 1974; Purnell and Gregg, 1975).

Perez-Reyes et al. in 1976 investigated the effect of intravenous infusion of six cannabinoids in healthy volunteers. Delta-8-THC, Δ-9-THC, 11-hydroxy-Δ-9-THC, cannabinol, cannabidiol, and 8-β-hydroxy-Δ-9-THC were tested on healthy subjects with normal intraocular pressure; Δ-8-THC, Δ-9-THC, and 11-hydroxy-THC caused the greatest reduction in pressure. Of these Δ-8-THC caused the largest decrease in intraocular pressure, with the least number of psychological side-effects.

In a preliminary study of 11 human glaucoma patients who smoked marijuana (1, 2, and 4 percent) or ingested Δ-9-THC (15 mg), intra-ocular pressure was lowered an average of 30 percent in 7 out of 11 patients (Hepler et al., 1976a). Another study showed that most patients had a decrease in intraocular pressure after ingestion of 15, 20, or 30 mg of Δ-9-THC and after smoking cannabis containing 1, 2, and 4 percent Δ-9-THC (Hepler et al., 1976b).

Ideally, the synthesis of a preparation that could be applied topically to the eye would be most desirable for humans, because this would allow for self-administration. However, initial studies in humans with a topical preparation of Δ-9-THC have not shown a consistent effect on intraocular pressure (Merritt et al., 1981). More work needs to be done on this possibility.

Animal Studies

While animal studies have supported the observation that Δ-9-THC lowers intraocular pressure after oral and topical administration in rabbits (Green et al., 1977a,b; 1978), and after intravenous adminis-tration in the cat (Innemee et al., 1979), the reduction in intra-ocular pressure is not completely understood. It may result in part from a central nervous system effect, and in part through action on the adrenergic system in the eye, probably mediated by the neuro-transmitter norepinephrine.

Side-Effects

Marijuana and Δ-9-THC given orally, intravenously, or in cigarettes to control glaucoma cause systemic side-effects, such as increase in heart rate, decrease in blood pressure, and psychotropic effects. Some of these side-effects are significant enough to pose problems, particularly in patients with glaucoma, who are usually elderly. But on the other hand, some of these effects may disappear as tolerance (decreased response with repeated use) develops.

Tolerance to the Intraocular Pressure Reducing Effect

No tolerance was detected to the ocular effects of cannabis in rabbits after 1 year's topical instillation of the synthetic cannabinoids SP-1, SP-106, and SP-204 (Green and Kim, 1977; Green et al., 1977b). Hepler et al. (1976b) noted a ceiling effect in humans, in that the smoking of 22 cannabis cigarettes did not result in a significant decrease in eyeball pressure as compared with a subject who smoked only 2 cigarettes. The area of tolerance will need further study, especially if a cannabinoid preparation with a satisfactorily high ratio of therapeutic to side-effects can be found.

Summary

Cannabis, Δ-9-THC, other cannabinoid derivatives, and their synthetics, reduce intraocular pressure in humans when smoked, or given intravenously or orally. However, there are systemic side-effects as well as psychotropic effects that are of concern. It is not yet clear whether an effective topical preparation can be developed that will not have these side-effects. Future work should determine whether synthetic cannabinoids or cannabinoid analogues can be found that will be effective in treating glaucoma without causing side-effects.

ANTIEMETIC ACTION

Certain cancer chemotherapeutic agents regularly produce nausea and vomiting after oral or intravenous administration. Those that are most severe in that respect are cisplatin, actinomycin D, adriamycin, cyclophosphamide, methotrexate, and the nitrosoureas. Other anti-cancer compounds may produce nausea less regularly or in less marked fashion.

Because cancer chemotherapy now can produce increased survival in patients with some neoplasms (recurrent or metastatic breast cancer, small cell carcinoma of the lung, ovarian cancer, and others) and substantial cure rates in several (acute lymphoblastic leukemia, Hodgkins disease, germ cell tumors of the testis, etc.) nausea and vomiting that interfere with patients' willingness to continue therapy can be a life-threatening side-effect. Even for those willing to endure the symptoms, they can be extremely unpleasant and debilitating.

Established antiemetics (prochlorperazine and other phenothia-zines) are not very effective against drug-induced emesis, and there is a need for new and more reliable antiemetic agents. Metoclopra-mide, a derivative of procainamide, has recently been shown to be more effective than prochlorperazine in certain situations and seems promising (Gralla et al., 1981).

The suggestion that cannabis might have some useful antiemetic activity in this setting arose about 1973, when patients receiving intensive chemotherapy for acute leukemia observed that their "social" use of cannabis appeared to reduce their customary nausea and vomiting.

Clinical Investigations

Several controlled studies have been reported. In one of the early ones (Sallan et al., 1975), Δ-9-THC in 15- or 20-mg doses by mouth was compared with a placebo in a randomized double-blind crossover trial in 22 patients whose nausea and vomiting had been shown refractory to other antiemetics. In 14 of 20 courses of treatment, patients obtained "complete or partial relief" with Δ-9-THC; in none of 22 courses did patients report benefit with the placebo. It was observed that the antiemetic effect of Δ-9-THC occurred only in association with the "high," and it was necessary to maintain the "high" in order to maintain the antiemetic effect.

In another controlled trial (Chang et al., 1979), 14 of 15 patients with osteogenic sarcoma treated with high-dose methotrexate had less nausea and vomiting with Δ-9-THC than with the placebo. In that study, patients with other tumors being treated with cytoxan and adriamycin did not respond as well. That report and others like it suggested that the antiemetic effect of Δ-9-THC against those chemotherapeutic agents that are moderate in their emetic potential (e.g., methotrexate) was pronounced, but that Δ-9-THC was less effective against those agents with severe emetic properties. In a similar study (Lucas and Laszlo, 1980), 38 of 53 patients with nausea and vomiting refractory to other antiemetics reported good results with Δ-9-THC. Among the failures were those treated with cisplatin, which has been characterized as one of the most emetic agents used in cancer chemotherapy.

In comparison with prochlorperazine, Δ-9-THC has also been reported to be more effective in preventing nausea and vomiting (Ekert et al., 1979; Sallan et al., 1980).

In a larger study (Frytak et al., 1979), of 116 patients treated with 5-fluouracil and methyl-CCNU, Δ-9-THC was said to be no more effective than prochlorperazine. In that study, in which nearly all patients were older than those in the other reported trials, the majority of patients considered the other side-effects of Δ-9-THC so unpleasant that they preferred either prochlorparazine or the placebo.

Another cannabinoid, a synthetic, nabilone, has been provided to several investigators for evaluation an an antiemetic agent; it has been licensed for use in Canada for treatment of nausea associated with cancer treatment. In the largest clinical study to date (Herman et al., 1979), nabilone was compared with prochlorperazine in a double-blind crossover trial. It was found more effective than prochlorperazine. The patients in that study preferred nabilone to prochlorperazine; the predominant side-effects were somnolence, dry mouth, and dizziness. Hallucinations occurred in a few patients. Euphoria of the type associated with cannabis was infrequent in that study. However, a study in dogs has revealed previously unrecognized late neurologic effects of nabilone at high doses (Archer et al., 1981). Monkeys and rats did not show similar toxic effects with long-term administration of nabilone (Archer et al., 1981), and further studies will be necessary to clarify the safety of this new agent.

Levonantradol is yet another synthetic cannabinoid, related to Δ-9-THC, which has been shown in preliminary clinical studies to have antiemetic action in patients with refractory chemotherapy-induced emesis (Diasio et al., 1981).

Uncontrolled Use of Δ-9-THC

In response to public and political pressures, the National Cancer Institute, the United States Drug Enforcement Agency, and the Food and Drug Administration have agreed to a program whereby the National Cancer Institute is making Δ-9-THC available through the pharmacies of approximately 500 teaching hospitals and cancer centers to physicians who wish to use Δ-9-THC in treating the nausea and vomiting of patients receiving cancer chemotherapy. This broad, uncontrolled program, in which no data other than the reporting of severe reactions are to be collected, may make it extremely difficult to obtain continuing valid evaluations of the effectiveness of Δ-9-THC in the management of nausea and vomiting due to cancer chemotherapy. Although the extent of use of Δ-9-THC under this program is difficult to evaluate, informal communication with the National Cancer Institute indicates that Δ-9-THC has been supplied in substantial quantities to several hundred hospital pharmacies. The problem is further complicated by the fact that the legislatures of 23 states have authorized the use of cannabis by any physician for the management of nausea and vomiting due to cancer chemotherapy. It is expected that little reliable information will be derived from such use.

Summary

There seems little doubt that Δ-9-THC and other cannabinoids are active against the severe nausea and vomiting produced by cancer chemotherapeutic agents. The extent of this activity, its relation to other antiemetics, and its relation to the other effects of the cannabinoids have not yet been accurately determined.

Cannabis leaf, smoked or eaten, is also antiemetic but its activity has been even less well determined than that of Δ-9-THC. Studies with other synthetic cannabinoids have barely begun and much remains to be learned in this field.

APPETITE STIMULANT

It has been stated by "social" users that the smoking of cannabis increases appetite. On that basis, there have been sporadic attempts to use it in patients with advanced cancer to overcome their customary debilitating weight loss.

In several of the studies in which Δ-9-THC was used as an antiemetic in patients receiving cancer chemotherapy, they were reported to have increased appetite and food intake. At this time, it is not certain whether that increase was due merely to relief of nausea and vomiting or to stimulation of appetite. One comparison of habitual marijuana users and controls matched for age and educational background showed increased caloric intake and weight gain among the users (Greenberg, et al., 1976). Furthermore, a double-blind controlled study (Hollister, 1971) of smokers of cannabis or placebo cigarettes provided with unlimited quantities of a high-caloric beverage indicated an increase in caloric consumption in those using cannabis compared with those using the placebo; however, the variability was very large and there was some question that cannabis could be considered a clinically significant appetite stimulant.

In another study of the psychological effects of Δ-9-THC in patients with advanced cancer, it was observed that Δ-9-THC appeared to stimulate appetite and retard weight loss (Regelson et al., 1976). In that study many patients refused to complete the 2-week trial because of unacceptable side-effects from Δ-9-THC.

The evidence to date suggests that there may be some influence of cannabis on appetite. However, it is not possible to separate that from the effect on nausea and vomiting. Further studies are in progress in cancer patients whose course is not complicated by nausea and vomiting.

ANTICONVULSANT ACTION

A large number of animal studies have been conducted using cannabis as an anticonvulsant. These can be divided into several categories. The first to be discussed will be maximal electroshock seizures (MES)* both in the rat and mouse (Loewe and Goodman, 1947; Sofia et al., 1971; Fujimoto, 1972; Consroe and Man, 1973; Karler et al., 1973; Chesher and Jackson, 1974; Karler et al., 1974; McCaughran et al., 1974; Karler and Turkanis, 1976; Consroe and Wolkin, 1977; Turkanis et al., 1977). In these studies there is a clear dose-response effect in the protection to MES conferred by cannabinol (CBN) and cannabidiol (CBD). Tolerance to the effect has frequently been reported. However, the tolerance noted with cannabinoids is similar to that seen with phenytoin (DPH). Further, even though tolerance to phenytoin develops with MES, this has not been shown to

---

*Electrical shock of maximum intensity to cause a major seizure.

be a clinically significant phenomenon. In these studies it is generally found that CBN is less effective against MES and against audiogenic seizures, the latter produced in rodents by loud noise, than CBD. In addition, Turkanis et al. (1977) have emphasized the fact that CBD acts more like DPH than other anticonvulsants and hence would be expected to be effective against major seizures rather than against minor seizures.

There is also extensive animal literature that CBN and CBD will protect against electrically induced, minimal (kindling) seizures (Corcoran et al., 1973; Fried and McIntyre, 1973; Izquierdo et al., 1973; Turkanis et al., 1977, 1979). Reduction of seizures produced by subcortical electrical stimulation in the cat has been reported (Wada et al., 1973). There appears to be much less effect on pentylenetetrazol-induced seizures (Consroe and Man, 1973; Turkanis et al., 1979). Any effect of CBN and CBD on such seizures occurs with maximal toxic doses (Turkanis et al., 1974). Protection against audiogenic seizures (Consroe et al., 1973) and against reflex seizures in the gerbil (Cox et al., 1975) have been reported.

Human studies are largely anecdotal and conflicting. There is one study by Cunha et al. (1980) in which 15 patients suffering from partial complex epilepsy with a temporal focus were randomly divided into two groups. Each patient received, in a double-blind procedure, 200-300 mg of CBD or placebo daily. The drugs were administered for as long as 4 1/2 months. Throughout the study, clinical and laboratory examinations, electroencephalograms, and electrocardiograms were performed at 15- to 30-day intervals. The patients continued their anticonvulsant medications taken before entering the study, on which all them had previously experienced uncontrolled seizures. All patients tolerated CBD well, and there were no signs of toxicity or serious side-effects. Four of the 8 CBD subjects remained nearly free of convulsions during CBD treatment and 3 other patients demonstrated partial improvement in their clinical condition. Cannabidiol was ineffective in 1 patient. The placebo group showed no alteration of seizure frequency. A series of 8 healthy volunteers given CBD showed no effects of the drug.

Summary

There is substantial evidence from animal studies to indicate that cannabinoids are effective in blocking both kindling seizures and MES, and this is particularly true for CBD. MES is a standard testing procedure for evaluation of anticonvulsant drugs. This is strong support for further investigation into the utility of CBD in human epilepsy. The one available carefully controlled human study is in accord with this review.

MUSCLE RELAXANT ACTION

There are widespread, anecdotal reports that cannabis is effective in relieving muscle spasm or spasticity. Petro (1980) has reported such effects in two cases and has carried out a double-blind study of the administration of Δ-9-THC on spasticity (Petro and Ellenberger, 1981). They reported that 10 mg of Δ-9-THC significantly reduced spasticity by clinical measurement and that quadriceps electromyograms demonstrated a decrease in interference pattern in four patients with primarily extensor spasticity. These are preliminary observations, but they suggest that further and more rigorous investigations of the use of cannabinoids in spasticity should be suggested to test their therapeutic effectiveness.

ANTIASTHMATIC EFFECT

Intensive, chronic smoking of concentrated cannabis produces several adverse effects on the airways, including mild bronchoconstriction. But acute smoking of cannabis as well as the ingestion of Δ-9-THC produces bronchodilation in normals and in subjects with chronic, clinically stable bronchial asthma of minimal to moderate severity (Tashkin et al., 1974). These bronchodilator effects were also investigated in individuals in whom an asthmatic attack was induced experimentally by exercise or methalcholine (Tashkin et al., 1975). Immediately after the development of bronchospasm, subjects smoked a cigarette containing 500 mg of cannabis assayed at either 1 or 2 percent Δ-9-THC.

Methalcholine inhalation promptly caused significant broncho-constriction (an average decrease in airway conductance of 40-55 percent) and significant hyperinflation (mean increases in thoracic gas volume of 35-43 percent). After placebo smoking or saline inhalation, airway conductance increased only modestly, remaining significantly less than initial control values for 30 to 60 minutes, and thoracic gas volume decreased only gradually, remaining significantly increased for 15 minutes. However, after 2 percent cannabis, and after isoproterenol, there was a prompt return of airway conductance and thoracic gas volume to control values.

Exercise in the asthma-prone individual resulted in average decreases in airway conductance of 30-39 percent and average increase in thoracic gas volume of 25-35 percent. After placebo or saline, there was only a gradual return to control values during 30-60 minutes, but after cannabis, airway conductance and thoracic gas volume returned promptly to preexercise values. Four of the subjects who had previously used cannabis could detect pleasurable sensations after smoking cannabis, which distinguished these effects from those of the placebo cigarette. In that sense these experiments were not strictly blind. The four subjects who had no previous experience with cannabis did not experience any central nervous system effects but did note mild somolence or light-headedness after cannabis. The results of this study suggest that any bronchial irritant effects of placebo cannabis smoke were not sufficient to aggravate or perpetuate existing acute bronchospasm to an extent greater than that which might result from the irritant effect of inhaled saline. The results also demonstrate that inhaled Δ-9-THC causes a prompt and complete sustained reversal of methacholine-induced bronchospasm and correction of the associated hyperinflation. These effects were not significantly different from those observed after isoproterenol, although there was a tendency toward a greater degree of bronchial dilation after isoproterenol. Similarly, after inhalation of Δ-9-THC, there was a prompt return of airway conductance and thoracic gas volume during exercise-induced bronchospasm to the preexercise value. After exercise the effects of 10 mg Δ-9-THC was not as efficacious as 1.25 mg isoproterenol.

The way in which Δ-9-THC induces bronchial dilation has not been determined, but previous studies have shown that this effect is not mediated by beta-adrenergic stimulation or inhibition of muscarine receptors (Shapiro et al., 1973). A vagolytic mechanism is possible, as suggested by other studies carried out on the dog salivary gland (Cavero et al., 1972) and on guinea pig ileum (Gill et al., 1970).

Although ingestion of Δ-9-THC in a sesame oil vehicle has produced bronchodilation in asthmatic patients (Tashkin et al., 1974), less dilation was noted than after smaller doses of Δ-9-THC delivered by smoking. Its significant bronchodilator effect notwithstanding, Δ-9-THC does not appear to be suitable for that therapeutic use, because of its psychotropic effects and possibly other side-effects. However, other cannabinoid compounds such as cannabinol and cannabidiol do not produce the central nervous system effects of tachycardia characteristic of cannabis (Hollister, 1973) and deserve further investigation for possible bronchodilator activity.

ANTIANXIETY EFFECT

Users of cannabis have often reported that the drug produces feelings of relaxation and calmness, and some have reported its use to reduce anxiety. A problem with evaluating cannabis as an antianxiety drug, however, is that some subjects report increased anxiety or panic after using cannabis (see Chapter 6). For example, Regelson et al. (1976) found less tension and apprehension in cancer patients after cannabis use; but 6 of 50 subjects receiving Δ-9-THC reported such side-effects as severe dizziness, confused thinking, dissociation, and concern over loss of sanity. In normals, Pillard et al. (1974) found no effects of cannabis on experimentally induced anxiety. Nabilone, a synthetic cannabinoid, was found to reduce experimentally induced anxiety in normal volunteers but it was less effective than diazepam (Nakano et al., 1978). Nabilone was found to be more effective than placebo in patients with psychoneurotic anxiety (Fabre et al., 1978).

There are very few studies of cannabis effects on anxiety. There is no indication at this time that cannabis or nabilone are more effective or reliable than currently available antianxiety medication.

ANTIDEPRESSANT EFFECT

Regelson et al. (1976) reported a significant reduction in self-rated depressive symptoms in cancer patients treated with Δ-9-THC. However, in a carefully controlled trial with four bipolar and four unpolar depressed patients, Kotin et al. (1973) found no anti-depressant activity.

ANALGESIC ACTION

Several animal models have been used to show analgesic effects of cannabis and its analogues (for example, Grunfeld and Edery, 1969; Sofia et al., 1973). Human studies have been conflicting. Milstein et al. (1975) found increase in tolerance to experimentally induced pain after smoking cannabis, while Hill et al. (1974) were unable to detect effects using a different kind of experimental pain. Noyes et al. (1976) found a reduction in pain reports by cancer patients given oral Δ-9-THC; Regelson et al. (1976) also studied cancer patients and found no significant changes in pain after Δ-9-THC.

Those subjects who show analgesic effects of cannabis also show other pharmacological effects such as mental clouding. The literature does not indicate a specific effect of cannabis on pain pathways nor does it suggest that cannabis is likely to be more effective than currently available analgesics.

ALCOHOLISM

Cannabis has been proposed as a treatment for alcoholism (Scher, 1971) based upon case reports and on the observation that cannabis and alcohol were generally not used together. A systematic evaluation (Rosenberg et al., 1978) failed to find cannabis useful in alcoholism. Moreover, recent surveys (see Chapter 2) indicate that currently the abuse of cannabis and alcohol are frequently combined.

OPIATE WITHDRAWAL

Early clinical reports suggested that cannabis might be useful in suppressing the symptoms of opiate withdrawal (Birch, 1889; Thompson and Proctor, 1953). Recently a series of animal studies (Hine et al., 1975a,b; Bhargava, 1976) have found that Δ-9-THC suppresses many of the behavioral manifestations of withdrawal precipitated by naloxone in morphine dependent rodents. This effect is enhanced by cannabidiol (CBD) (Hine et al., 1975a,b), but CBD is not effective alone.

There are no reports of systematic evaluations of cannabis as a treatment of opiate withdrawal in human beings. The animal studies do not present evidence that cannabis is likely to be more effective than currently available treatments for opiate withdrawal.

ANTITUMOR ACTION

There is very little information about the effects of cannabis on neoplasms. In one study (Harris et al., 1976), minor effects were seen on the Lewis Lung Tumor but not in L1210 leukemia. In another study (White et al., 1976), it was found that Δ-9-THC inhibited tumor DNA replication somewhat. In that same study, cannabidiol appeared to have a growth enhancing effect on the Lewis Lung Tumor. These limited studies do not support a view that Δ-9-THC has a useful effect in inhibiting tumor growth.

SUMMARY

Cannabis and its derivatives have shown promise in the treatment of a variety of disorders. The evidence is most impressive in glaucoma, where their mechanism of action appears to be different from the standard drugs; in asthma, where they approach isoproterenol in effectiveness; and in the nausea and vomiting of cancer chemotherapy, where they compare favorably with phenothiazines. Smaller trials have suggested cannabis might also be useful in seizures, spasticity, and other nervous system disorders. Effective doses usually produce psychotropic and cardiovascular effects and can be troublesome, particularly in older patients.

Although marijuana has not been shown unequivocally superior to any existing therapy for any of these conditions, several important aspects of its therapeutic potential should be appreciated. First, its mechanisms of action and its toxicity in several diseases are different from those of drugs now being used to treat those conditions; thus, combined use with other drugs might allow greater therapeutic efficacy without cumulative toxicity. Second, the differences in action suggest new approaches to understanding both the diseases and the drugs used to treat them. Last, there may be an opportunity to synthesize derivatives of marijuana that offer better therapeutic ratios than marijuana itself.

RECOMMENDATIONS FOR RESEARCH

The committee believes that the therapeutic potential of cannabis and its derivatives and synthetic analogues warrants further research along the lines described in this chapter. There also may be significant heuristic benefits to be derived from the study of the biological mechanisms by which these compounds act.

Some therapeutic promise seems to be offered by synthetic cannabinoid analogues. The committee recommends that particular attention be paid to the treatment of chemotherapy-induced nausea and vomiting in cancer patients because current management of this important and widespread problem is inadequate and preliminary studies suggest that cannabinoids may have some special advantage. Cannabinoids or their analogues also may find a place in the management of resistant glaucoma, of severe intractable asthma, and of certain forms of seizures that are resistant to standard therapy. Continued carefully contracted clinical trials in these areas seem worthwhile at this time, as do studies of the usefulness of cannabinoids in the treatment of muscle spasticity.

REFERENCES

Archer, R.A., Hanasono, G.K., Lemberger, L., and Sullivan, H.R. Update on nabilone research: the relationship of metabolism to toxicity in dogs, pp. 119-127. In Poster, D.S., Penta, J.S., and Bruno, S. (eds.) Treatment of Cancer Chemotherapy Induced Nausea and Vomiting. New York: Moser Publishing Co., 1981.

Bhargava, H.N. Effect of some cannabinoids on naloxone-precipitated abstinence in morphine-dependent mice. Psychopharmacology 49:267-270, 1976.

Birch, E.A. The use of Indian hemp in the treatment of chronic chloral and chronic opium poisoning. Lancet 1:625, 1889.

Cavero, I., Buckley, J.P., and Jandhyala, B.S. Parasympatholytic activity of (-)-delta-9-transtetrahydrocannabinol in mongrel dogs. Eur. J. Pharmacol. 19:301-304, 1972.

Chang, A.E., Shiling, D.J., Stillman, R.C., et al. Delta-9-tetrahydrocannabinol as an antiemetic in cancer patients receiving high-dose methotrexate: A prospective, randomized evaluation. Ann. Int. Med. 91:819-824, 1979.

Chesher, G.B. and Jackson, D.M. Anticonvulsant effects of cannabinoids in mice: Drug interactions within cannabinoids and cannabinoid interactions with phenytoin. Psychopharmacologia 37:255-264, 1974.

Consroe, P.F. and Man, D.P. Effects of delta-8- and delta-9-tetrahydrocannabinol on experimentally induced seizures. Life Sci. 13:429-439, 1973.

Consroe, P. and Wolkin, A. Cannabidiol--Antiepileptic drug comparisons and interactions in experimentally induced seizures in rats. J. Pharmacol. Exp. Ther. 201:26-32, 1977.

Consroe, P.F., Man, D.P., Chin, L., and Picchioni, A.L. Reduction of audiogenic seizure by delta-8- and delta-9-tetrahydrocannabinols. J. Pharm. Pharmacol. 25:764-765, 1973.

Corcoran, M.E., McCaughran, J.A., Jr., and Wada, J.A. Acute antiepileptic effects of delta-9-tetrahydrocannabinol in rats with kindled seizures. Exp. Neurol. 40:471-483, 1973.

Cox, B., ten Ham, M., Loskota, W.J., and Lomax, P. The anticonvulsant activity of cannabinoids in seizure sensitive gerbils. Proc. West. Pharmacol. Soc. 18:154-157, 1975.

Cunha, J.M., Carlini, E.A., Pereira, A.E., et al. Chronic administration of cannabidiol to healthy volunteers and epileptic patients. Pharmacology 21:175-185, 1980.

Diasio, R.B., Ettinger, D.S., and Satterwhite, B.E. Oral levonantradol in the treatment of chemotherapy-induced emesis: Preliminary observations. J. Clin. Pharmacol. 21:81S-85S, 1981.

Ekert, H., Waters, K.D., Jurk, I.H., et al. Amelioration of cancer chemotherapy-induced nausea and vomiting by delta-9-tetrahydrocannabinol. Med. J. Aust. 2:657-659, 1979.

Fabre, L.F., McLendon, D.M., and Stark, P. Nabilon, a cannabinoid, in the treatment of anxiety: An open-label and double-blind study. Curr. Ther. Res. 24:161-169, 1978.

Fried, P.A. and McIntyre, D.C. Electrical and behavioral attenuation of the anti-convulsant properties of delta-9-THC following chronic administrations. Psychopharmacologia 31:215-227, 1973.

Frytak, S., Moertel, C.G., O'Fallon, J.R., et al. Delta-9-tetrahydrocannabinol as an antiemetic for patients receiving cancer chemotherapy: A comparison with prochlorperazine and a placebo. Ann. Intern. Med. 91:825-830, 1979.

Fujimoto, J.M. Modification of the effects of delta-9-tetrahydrocannabinol by phenobarbital pretreatment in mice. Toxicol. Appl. Pharmacol. 23:623-634, 1972.

Gill, E.W., Paton, W.D.M., and Pertwee, R.G. Preliminary experiments on the chemistry and pharmacology of cannabis. Nature 228:134-136, 1970.

Gralla, R.J., Itri, L.M., Pisko, S.E., et al. Antiemetic efficacy of high-dose metoclopramide: Randomized trials with placebo and prochlorperazine in patients with chemotherapy-induced nausea and vomiting. N. Engl. J. Med. 305:905-909, 1981.

Green, K. The ocular effects of cannabinoids, pp. 175-215. In Zadunaisky, J.A. (ed.) Current Topics in Eye Research. New York: Academic Press, 1979.

Green, K. and Kim, K. Acute dose response of intraocular pressure to topical and oral cannabinoids. Proc. Soc. Exp. Biol. Med. 154:228-231, 1977.

Green, K., Bigger, J.F., Kim, K., and Bowman, K. Cannabinoid penetration and chronic effects in the eye. Exp. Eye Res. 24:197-205, 1977a.

Green, K., Kim, K., Wynn, H., and Shimp, R.G. Intraocular pressure, organ weights, and the chronic use of cannabinoid derivatives in rabbits for one year. Exp. Eye Res. 25:465-471, 1977b.

Green, K., Wynn, H., and Bowman, K.A. A comparison of topical cannabinoids on intraocular pressure. Exp. Eye Res. 27:239-246, 1978.

Greenberg, I., Kuehnle, J., Mendelson, J.H., and Bernstein, J.G. Effects of marihuana use on body weight and calorie intake in humans. Psychopharmacology 49:79-84, 1976.

Grunfeld, Y. and Edery, H. Psychopharmacological activity of some substances extracted from cannabis sativa L (hashish). Electroencephalogr. Clin. Neurophysiol. 27:219-220, 1969.

Harris, L.S., Munson, A.E., and Carchman, R.A. Antitumor properties of cannabinoids, pp. 749-762. In Braude, M.C. and Szara, S. (eds.) Pharmacology of Marihuana. New York: Raven Press, 1976.

Hepler, R.S. and Frank, I.M. Marijuana smoking and intraocular pressure. JAMA 217:1392, 1971.

Hepler, R.S., Frank, I.M., and Ungerleider, J.T. Pupillary constriction after marijuana smoking. Am. J. Ophthalmol. 74:1185-1190, 1972.

Hepler, R.S., Frank, I.M., and Petrus, R. Ocular effects of marijuana smoking, pp. 815-824. In Braude, M.C. and Szara, S. (eds.) Pharmacology of Marihuana. New York: Raven Press, 1976a.

Hepler, R.S. and Petrus, R.J. Experiences with administration of marijuana to glaucoma patients, pp. 63-75. In Cohen, S. and Stillman, R.C. (eds.) The Therapeutic Potential of Marihuana. New York: Plenum Medical Book Company, 1976b.

Herman, T.S., Einhorn, L.H., Jones, S.E., et al. Superiority of nabilone over prochlorperazine as an antiemetic in patients receiving cancer chemotherapy. N. Engl. J. Med. 300:1295-1297, 1979.

Hill, S.Y., Goodwin, D.W., Schwin, R., and Powell, B. Marijuana: CNS depressant or excitant? Am. J. Psychiatry 131:313-315, 1974.

Hine, B., Friedman, E., Torrelio, M., and Gershon, S. Tetrahydrocannabinol-attenuated abstinence and induced rotation in morphine-dependent rats: Possible involvement of dopamine. Neuropharmacology 14:607-610, 1975a.

Hine, B., Friedman, E., Torrelio, M., and Gershon, S. Morphine-dependent rats: Blockade of precipitated abstinence by tetrahydrocannabinol. Science 187:443-445, 1975b.

Hollister, L.E. Hunger and appetite after single doses of marihuana, alcohol, and dextroamphetamine. Clin. Pharmacol. Ther. 12:44-49, 1971.

Hollister, L.E. Cannabidiol and cannabinol in man. Experientia 29:825-826, 1973.

Innemee, H.C., Hermans, A.J.M., and Van Zwieten, P.A. The influence of delta-9-tetrahydrocannabinol on intraocular pressure in the anaesthetized cat. Doc. Ophthalmol. 48:235-241, 1979.

Izquierdo, I., Orsingher, O.A., and Berardi, A.C. Effect of cannabidiol and of other cannabis sativa compounds on hippocampal seizure discharges. Psychopharmacologia 28:95-102, 1973.

Karler, R. and Turkanis, S.A. The development of tolerance and "reverse tolerance" to the anticonvulsant activity of delta-9-tetrahydrocannabinol and cannabidiol, pp. 299-311. In Braude, M.C. and Szara, S. (eds.) Pharmacology of Marihuana. New York: Raven Press, 1976.

Karler, R., Cely, W., and Turkanis, S.A. The anticonvulsant activity of cannabidiol and cannabinol. Life Sci. 13:1527-1531, 1973.

Karler, R., Cely, W., and Turkanis, S.A. Anticonvulsant properties of delta-9-tetrahydrocannabinol and other cannabinoids. Life Sci. 15:931-947, 1974.

Kotin, J., Post, R.M., and Goodwin, F.K. Δ-9-Tetrahydrocannabinol in depressed patients. Arch. Gen. Psychiatry 28:345-348, 1973.

Loewe, S. and Goodman, L.S. Anticonvulsant action of marihuana-active substances. Fed. Proc. 6:352, 1947.

Lucas, V.S. and Laszlo, J. Delta-9-tetrahydrocannabinol for refractory vomiting induced by cancer chemotherapy. JAMA 243:1241-1243, 1980.

McCaughran, J.A., Corcoran, M.E., and Wada, J.A. Anticonvulsant activity of delta-8 and delta-9-tetrahydrocannabinol in rats. Pharmacol. Biochem. Behav. 2:227-233, 1974.

Merritt, J.C. Perry, D.D., Russell, D.N., and Jones, B.F. Tropical Δ-9-tetrahydrocannabinol and aqueous dynamics in glaucoma. J. Clin. Pharmacol. 21:467S-471S, 1981.

Milstein, S.L., MacCannell, K., Karr, G., and Clark, S. Marijuana-produced changes in pain tolerance. Experienced and nonexperienced subjects. Int. Pharmacopsychiat. 10:177-182, 1975.

Nakano, S., Gillespie, H.K., and Hollister, L.E. A model for evaluation of antianxiety drugs with the use of experimentally induced stress: Comparison of nabilon and diazepam. Clin. Pharmacol. Ther. 23:54-62, 1978.

National Society to Prevent Blindness. Facts and Figures, 1980.

Noyes, R., Brunk, S.F., Avery, D.H., and Canter, A. Psychologic effects of oral delta-9-tetrahydrocannabinol in advanced cancer patients. Compr. Psychiatry 17:641-646, 1976.

Perez-Reyes, M., Wagner, D., Wall, M.E., and Davis, K.H. Intravenous administration of cannabinoids and intraocular pressure, pp. 829-832. In Braude, M.C. and Szara, S. (eds.) Pharmacology of Marihuana. New York: Raven Press, 1976.

Petro, D.J. Marihuana as a therapeutic agent for muscle spasm or spasticity. Psychosomatics 21:81-85, 1980.

Petro, D.J. and Ellenberger, C. Treatment of human spasticity with Δ-9-tetrahydrocannabinol. J. Clin. Pharmacol. 21:413S-416S, 1981.

Pillard, R.C., McNair, D.M., and Fisher, S. Does marijuana enhance experimentally induced anxiety? Psychopharmacologia 40:205-210, 1974.

Purnell, W.D. and Gregg, J.M. Delta-9-tetrahydrocannabinol, euphoria and intraocular pressure in man. Ann. Ophthalmol. 7:921-923, 1975.

Regelson, W., Butler, J.R., Shulz, J., et al. Delta-9-tetrahydrocannabinol as an effective antidepressant and appetite-stimulating agent in advanced cancer patients, pp. 763-776. In Braude, M.C. and Szara, S. (eds.) Pharmacology of Marihuana. New York: Raven Press, 1976.

Rosenberg, C.M., Gerrein, J.R., and Schnell, C. Cannabis in the treatment of alcoholism. J. Stud. Alcohol 39:155-1958, 1978.

Sallan, S.E., Zinberg, N.E., and Frei, E. Antiemetic effect of delta-9-tetrahydrocannabinol in patients receiving cancer chemotherapy. N. Engl. J. Med. 293:795-797, 1975.

Sallan, S.E., Cronin, C., Zelen, M., and Zinberg, N.E. Antiemetics in patients receiving chemotherapy for cancer: A randomized comparison of delta-9-tetrahydrocannabinol and prochlorperazine. N. Engl. J. Med. 302:135-138, 1980.

Scher, J. Marijuana as an agent in rehabilitating alcoholics. Am. J. Psychiatry 127:971-972, 1971.

Shapiro, D. The ocular mainfestations of the cannabinols. Ophthalmologica 168:366-369, 1974.

Shapiro, B.J., Tashkin, D.P., and Frank, I.M. Mechanism of increased specific airway conductance with marijuana smoking in healthy young men. Ann. Int. Med. 78:832-833, 1973.

Sofia, R.D., Solomon, T.A., and Barry, H. The anticonvulsant activity in delta-9-tetrahydrocannabinol in mice. Pharmacologist 13:246, 1971.

Sofia, R.D., Nalepa, S.D., Harakal, J.J., and Vassar, H.B. Anti-edema dna analgesic properties of Δ-9-tetrahyrocannabinol (THC). J. Pharmacol. Exp. Ther. 186:646-655, 1973.

Tashkin, D.P., Shapiro, B.J., and Frank, I.M. Acute effects of smoked marijuana and oral delta-9-tetrahydrocannabinol on specific airway conductance in asthmatic subjects. Am. Rev. Respir. Dis. 109:420-428, 1974.

Tashkin, D.P., Shapiro, B.J., Lee, Y.E., and Harper, C.E. Effects of smoked marijuana in experimentally induced asthma. Am. Rev. Respir. Dis. 112:377-386, 1975.

Thompson, L.J. and Proctor, R.C. The use of pyrahexyl in the treatment of alcoholic and drug withdrawal conditions. N.C. Med. J. 14:520-523, 1953.

Turkanis, S.A., Cely, W., Olsen, D.M., and Karler, R. Anticonvulsant properties of cannabidiol. Res. Commun. Chem. Pathol. Pharmacol. 8:231-246, 1974.

Turkanis, S.A., Chiu, P., Borys, H.K., and Karler, R. Influence of delta-9-tetrahydrocannabinol and cannabidiol on photically evoked after-discharge potentials. Psychopharmacology 52:207-212, 1977.

Turkanis, S.A., Smiley, K.A., Borys, H.K., et al. An electrophysiological analysis of the anticonvulsant action of cannabidiol on limbic seizures in conscious rats. Epilepsia 20:351-363, 1979.

Wada, J.A., Sato, M., and Corcoran, M.E. Antiepileptic properties of delta-9-tetrahydrocannabinol. Exp. Neurol. 39:157-165, 1973.

White, A.C., Munson, J.A., Munson, A.E., et al. Effects of delta-9-tetrahydrocannabinol in Lewis lung adenocarcinoma cells in tissue culture. J. Natl. Cancer Inst. 56:655-658, 1976.

8

FEDERAL SUPPORT OF
RESEARCH ON MARIJUANA

PRESENT SOURCES AND AMOUNTS OF SUPPORT

In this chapter the committee has examined sources and amounts of federal support for research on cannabis and the areas of research support. The committee has not analyzed the scientific substance of the work, nor has it examined the strategy of research support or reviewed current unpublished research.

The overall federal support for research on cannabis for the fiscal years 1977, 1978, and 1979 has averaged slightly more than $4 million per year in real dollars (Table 4). During these years, 11 federal agencies allocated funds for this purpose. Of these, the National Institute on Drug Abuse (NIDA) has been the principal agency, accounting for over four-fifths of the total, therefore, our analysis will focus primarily on this agency.

For fiscal years 1975 through 1980, NIDA's support of research on cannabis amounted to $4.5, $2.9, $3.9, $3.6, $3.5, and $3.8 million, respectively, in real dollars, but in constant 1981 dollars, corrected by the GNP deflator, the same figures were $7.0, $4.2, $5.4 $4.6, $4.2, and $4.1 (Table 5). Although the total research budget of this agency for those years increased by approximately $12 million (real dollars), the percent spent on cannabis declined from 14.2 to 8.2 (Table 5). During the same period, the total number of projects on cannabis supported by NIDA was reduced by approximately 50 percent; however, the cost per project increased from $42,700 to $71,400 (real dollars). This increased cost per project is still somewhat lower than the mean cost of all projects funded by the National Institutes of Health in 1980 (Leventhal, 1981).

Table 6 shows the NIDA extramural research programs for fiscal years 1975 through 1981, allocated according to the type of drug being studied. In FY 1975 research on cannabis was allocated only 13 percent of the total extramural budget, whereas narcotics and narcotic antagonists received more than 40 percent. Thereafter, the percentage devoted to cannabis declined, to a low of 8 percent in FY 1979, but started to rise again slightly in FY 1980 and FY 1981. In the last year, an estimated 11 percent of the budget was spent on cannabis research. The percent of the budget allocated to narcotics and narcotic antagonists has declined steadily, while the percentages

TABLE 4 Cannabis Research by Federal Agency: FY 1977-1979 (real dollars in thousands)

	Total (77) No. of grants	Funds	Percent	Total (78) No. of grants	Funds	Percent	Total (79) No. of grants	Funds	Percent
ADAMHA[b]									
NIDA	75	3,940	90	64	3,596	88	65	3,536	84
NIMH	8	167	4	8	214	5	7	207	5
NIAAA	2	8	a	5	85	2	6	122	3
NIH									
NCI	4	91	2	2	80	2	2	85	2
NEI	--	--	0	3	68	2	1	36	1
NICHD	--	--	0	1	13	a	1	15	a
NIRR	--	--	0	2	26	0	--	--	0
NIGMS	--	--	0	--	--	0	1	9	a
OTHER AGENCIES									
VA	7	52	1	6	26	1	8	25	1
DOT	5	55	1	1	--	a	2	104	2
USDA	1	41	1	-	--	0	1	85	2
TOTAL	102	4,354		92	4,106		94	4,202	

[a]less than 1 percent.

[b]

ADAMHA	Alcohol, Drug Abuse and Mental Health Administration
DHHS	Department of Health and Human Services
DOT	Department of Transportation
NCI	National Cancer Institute
NEI	National Eye Institute
NIAAA	National Institute on Alcohol Abuse and Alcoholism
NICHD	National Institute of Child Health and Human Development
NIDA	National Institute on Drug Abuse
NIGMS	National Institute of General Medical Sciences
NIH	National Institutes of Health
NIMH	National Institute of Mental Health
NIRR	National Institute of Research Resources
VA	Veterans Administration
USDA	Department of Agriculture

Source: Adapted from information provided by NIDA.

TABLE 5 Total Research and Research on Cannabis in NIDA Budget

	FY '73	FY '74	FY '75	FY '76	FY '77	FY '78	FY '79	FY '80	FY '81
Total NIDA research budget (real dollars, thousands)	31,600	34,000	34,046	33,760	33,994	33,986	42,930	45,972	40,400
Total NIDA research budget (constant 1981 dollars, thousands)	58,500	58,700	53,500	49,600	46,800	43,800	51,000	50,300	40,400
Cannabis research budget (real dollars, thousands)	a	a	4,483	2,853	3,940	3,596	3,536	3,788	a
Cannabis research budget (constant 1981 dollars, thousands)	a	a	7,043	4,191	5,421	4,636	4,201	4,144	a
Percent cannabis research	a	a	14.2	9.1	11.6	10.6	8.2	8.2	a
Total cannabis projects (real dollars, thousands)	a	a	105	82	75	64	65	53	a
Mean cannabis project cost (real dollars, thousands)	a	a	42.70	34.8	52.5	56.2	54.4	71.5b	a
Mean cannabis project cost (constant 1981 dollars, thousands)	a	a	67.1	51.1	72.3	72.5	64.6	78.2	a

[a] Data unavailable at present time.
[b] Mean NIH Project Cost (1980) was 105.

Source: Adapted from information provided by NIDA.

TABLE 6 NIDA Extramural Research Program, Distribution by Drug (real dollars in thousands)

Drug Class	FY 1975 Amount	%	FY 1976 Amount	%	FY 1977 Amount	%	FY 1978 Amount	%	FY 1979 Amount	%	FY 1980 Amount	%	FY 1981[a] Amount	%
Cannabis	4,104	13	3,694	12	3,532	11	3,114	10	3,263	8	3,683	9	4,500	11
Depressants	1,642	5	1,527	5	1,976	6	1,557	5	1,123	3	1,495	4	1,000	3
Hallucinogens	316	1	729	2	1,572	5	1,515	5	2,358	6	2,865	7	3,000	7
Narcotics	9,787	31	11,298	36	11,766	37	9,341	30	8,947	23	10,667	25	10,000	25
Narcotic antagonists	3,473	11	3,061	10	3,017	10	3,526	11	3,879	10	2,304	5	2,800	7
Stimulants	1,926	6	2,360	8	2,291	7	2,535	8	2,778	7	3,277	8	4,000	10
Volatiles/solvents	158	1	363	1	496	2	556	2	294	1	278	1	500	1
Tobacco	--	--	--	--	110	0	934	3	1,130	3	2,973	7	3,200	8
Endogenous substances	--	--	--	--	--	--	1,337	4	2,717	7	2,607	6	3,400	8
Polydrug, unspecified, other	10,169	32	8,166	26	6,731	22	6,723	22	12,286	32	11,875	28	8,008	20
TOTAL	31,575	100	31,198	100	31,491	100	31,138	100	38,775	100	42,024	100	40,408	100

[a]Estimate.

Source: Adapted from information provided by NIDA.

devoted to hallucinogens, stimulants, and "endogenous substances" have increased.

In FY '80, only $3,683,000 (9 percent) of the extramural budget was devoted to cannabis research. Almost as much was spent that year by NIDA on stimulants and on tobacco. For comparison, the National Cancer Institute's budget for its program "Smoking and Health" was $13.2 million in FY '80, of which $3.9 million was allocated for tobacco research (Little, 1981). The National Heart, Lung, and Blood Institute allocated $8.2 million to study the effects of cigarette smoking on the cardiovascular repiratory system (Hurd, 1981).

AREAS OF RESEARCH SUPPORT

Cannabis research essentially began in the late 1960s with a National Institute of Mental Health program to produce "pedigreed" cannabis for research investigators. NIDA, which was created in 1972, started with an extramural budget of $29.6 million and an intramural budget of $4.0 million for fiscal year 1973 (Ludford, 1981). In the early 1970s, NIDA's major thrusts were (a) supplying (to researchers) standardized marijuana of a known concentration of Δ-9-THC and of known genetic stock, (b) facilitating administrative mechanisms, and (c) attempting to understand the problem of drug abuse, e.g., how many people use the drug, what are the acute effects, and what are its implications (Petersen, 1981).

Recently, NIDA's emphasis has shifted to studying certain groups, e.g., children, adolescents, and pregnant women, especially with respect to the long-term effects of cannabis on these groups (Petersen, 1981). The NIDA program plan for fiscal year 1982 stresses that chronic and acute studies need to be conducted on the effects of cannabis and other drugs of abuse on women and adolescents, with a special emphasis on: (a) in-depth behavioral and biological studies of the amotivational syndrome ("burn-out"), and (b) the development of approaches to treatment. Also specifically targeted are studies of the effects on brain function and structure.

Table 7 presents the NIDA projects on cannabis for fiscal years 1978, 1979, and 1980 stratified by research goal. These research goals are defined in the footnote to the table. For fiscal years 1978, 1979, and 1980, most of the money devoted to research on cannabis (approximately $3 million annually) was spent in three areas: (1) hazards of cannabis use, (2) basic research, and (3) research support. This last goal includes the growth, processing, packaging, and distribution of cannabis, as well as the development of the Δ-9-THC capsule. It is instructive to compare this distribution of cannabis funds with the distribution of the total research funds of NIDA. In FY '80, research on hazards took only 12 percent of the total NIDA research budget, basic research 42 percent, and research support 19 percent (Pollin, 1981).

The allocation of funds, by research topic, for fiscal years 1978, 1979, and 1980 is presented in Table 8. The largest proportion of the funds has been allocated to two research topics: (1) drug

161

TABLE 7   NIDA Cannabis Projects by Research Goal: FY 1978-1980
(real dollars in thousands)

Goals	FY 1978	FY 1979	FY 1980
1. Epidemiology	238	54	61
2. Etiology	145	133	136
3. Prevention	77		48
4. Hazards	916	990	1,236
5. Therapeutic uses of cannabis	43	49	50
6. Treatment of cannabis abuse	11	2	82
7. Basic research	972	1,295	1,036
8. General research support	1,194	1,013	1,139
TOTAL	3,596	3,536	3,788

1.   Epidemiology--to determine the incidence, prevalence, trends, and distribution of drug abuse by sex, race, geographic origin, and other special characteristics.

2.   Etiology--to determine the etiologic factors associated with drug abuse, including those combinations of biological, psychological, and societal factors most associated with increased risk for misuse and/or abuse of drugs.

3.   Prevention--to develop and test new strategies and methods which might decrease, postpone, or modify drug-abusing behavior

4.   Hazards--to determine the hazards of drug abuse to the physical and mental health of the individual and its adverse effects on society.

5.   Therapeutic uses--to study the effectiveness and safety of cannabis in the treatment of various medical conditions.

6.   Treatment--to determine the most effective therapeutic procedures for reducing drug abuse including new and innovative treatment methods and development of more effective drugs to be used in treatment.

7.   Basic research--to advance basic knowledge of the pharmacology, biochemistry, and neurophysiology of drugs, the basic mechanisms involved in drug tolerance, and dependence and the underlying processes involved in addictive and/or habitual behaviors.

8.   Research support--to develop the methodological and support resources required to further drug abuse research; to provide for the publication and evaluation of research results, the analysis and supply of controlled substances, and the development of chemical methods to detect and assay drugs.

Source: Adapted from information provided by NIDA.

TABLE 8   NIDA Cannabinoid Projects by Research Topic: FY 1978-1980 (real dollars in thousands)

	FY 1978	FY 1979	FY 1980
Assay and models	482	302	268
Drug development, synthesis, and distribution	706	756	950
Psychophysiology	54	76	16
Performance (esp. driving)	193	111	76
Reproduction and development	491	864	849
Behavioral studies	124	62	15
Other drug effects/toxicity	397	347	440
Metabolism and pharmacokinetics	261	446	259
Immunology	69	85	--
Drug interactions	--	64	97
Chemistry	67	58	103
Mechanism of tolerance and dependence	285	174	134
Cultural/ethnic	195	45	69
Patterns and lifestyle	57	80	127
Crime/law	137	66	337
Abuse liability	76	--	48
TOTAL	3,594[a]	3,536	3,788

[a]Due to rounding of numbers, the total value is not exactly the same as in Table 7.

Source: Adapted from information provided by NIDA.

development, synthesis, and distribution; and (2) drug effects on reproduction and development.

Grants, Contracts, and Intramural Projects

Tables 9 through 11 compare the number of grants, contracts, and intramural projects on cannabis, as well as the funds expended by each agency for fiscal years 1977, 1978, and 1979. In each of these years, most of the extramural awards and most of the money involved investigator-initiated research grants. The ratio of grant to contract funds rose during this period from approximately 1.5 in FY '77 to almost 3.0 in FY '79. For NIDA as a whole, that ratio has consistently been much higher; in FY '79, for example, the funding of grants was more than five times that of contracts.

Support of investigator-initiated research grants requires that grant applications be approved by a peer review committee. In the peer review process, each approved grant is given a priority score based on scientific merit of the proposal (scaled from 100 to 500, with 100 the highest). This priority score determines the order in which available funds are dispersed. The award rate for all drug research supported by NIDA is shown in Table 12. The percentage of grants recommended for approval has increased slightly over recent years, as has the total number of grant applications. However, the percent of approved grants that has been funded has gone down sharply, as shown in the table. For FY '81 it is estimated that only 25 percent of all applicants were ultimately funded. The priority score at the 90th percentile of funded applications has also been declining, and in 1981 was estimated at 190. These data suggest that there has been no decline in the quality of funded grants--if anything, the quality has risen during the past few years.

The number of investigator-initiated projects has decreased slightly but still exceeds the number of contracts and intramural projects. Grants generally are for a period of 3 years (renewable on a year-to-year basis), with a maximum period of 5 years (Petersen, 1981). Contract projects are funded on a year-to-year basis and are mainly concerned with the growth, processing, packaging, and distribution of cannabis, as well as with the development of the Δ-9-THC capsule.* A few studies are conducted on toxicology and pharmacokinetics (Petersen, 1981). For fiscal years 1977, 1978, and 1979, the number of contracts has declined: 16, 14, and 10, respectively. However, the requests for proposals for fiscal years 1980 and 1981 have increased to 12 and 14, respectively (Ludford, 1981).

Intramural projects account for a small portion of the budget; for fiscal years 1977, 1978, and 1979, they have been declining.

---

*NIDA has requested that the NIH take over the cost and distribution of the drugs for clinical studies (Snyder, 1981).

TABLE 9 Cannabinoid Research by Agency: FY 1977
(real dollars in thousands)

	Grants		Contracts		Intramural		Total	
	No.	Funds	No.	Funds	No.	Funds	No.	Funds
ADAMHA								
NIDA	55	2,267	16	1,629	4	44	75	3,940
NIMH	8	167	--	--	--	--	8	167
NIAAA	2	8	--	--	--	--	2	8
NIH								
NCI	4	91	--	--	--	--	4	91
NEI	--	--	--	--	--	--	--	--
NCHD	--	--	--	--	--	--	--	--
NIRR	--	--	--	--	--	--	--	--
NIGMS	--	--	--	--	--	--	--	--
OTHER AGENCIES								
VA	--	--	--	--	7	52	7	52
DOT	--	--	2	55	--	--	2	55
USDA	--	--	--	--	1	41	1	41
TOTAL	69	2,533	18	1,684	12	137	99	4,354

Source: Adapted from information provided by NIDA.

SUMMARY OF FINDINGS

Total federal support for research on cannabis has been declining in real dollars over the past 3 years. Most of that support comes from the NIDA research budget, which allocates approximately 10 percent of its resources to this purpose. The current level of funding, under 4 million dollars, supports only about 50 extramural projects and represents only one-tenth of the total research program of NIDA. This decline in support has inexplicably occurred during a period when the concern of the public and of all levels of government seems to be rising. It cannot be explained by lack of interest in the field, for research grant applications have risen; neither can it be

TABLE 10 Cannabinoid Research By Agency: FY 1978
(real dollars in thousands)

	Grants		Contracts		Intramural		Total	
	No.	Funds	No.	Funds	No.	Funds	No.	Funds
ADAMHA								
NIDA	47	2,104	14	1,460	3	30	64	3,594
NIMH	5	158	--	--	3	56	8	214
NIAAA	5	85	--	--	--	--	5	85
NIH								
NCI	2	80	--	--	--	--	2	80
NEI	3	68	--	--	--	--	3	68
NCHD	1	13	--	--	--	--	1	13
NIRR	2	26	--	--	--	--	2	26
NIGMS	--	--	--	--	--	--	--	--
OTHER AGENCIES								
VA	--	--	--	--	6	26	6	26
DOT	--	--	1	a	--	--	1	a
USDA	--	--	--	--	--	--	--	--
TOTAL	65	2,534	15	1,460	12	112	92	4,106

a Indicates a funding level of less than $1000.

Source: Adapted from information provided by NIDA.

attributed to lack of scientific opportunity; for every area we have
studied, the committee has identified important questions that seem
amenable to new research efforts. (Many of these have been
enumerated in the preceding chapters.)

In FY '80, NIDA spent a nearly equal amount on stimulant drugs
and more than four times as much on narcotics and narcotic antagonists. Most of the cannabis research is devoted to three areas in
approximately equal amounts: (1) growth, processing and distribution;
(2) hazards of cannabis use; and (3) basic research. Three quarters
of all the federal research money devoted to cannabis goes to

TABLE 11 Cannabinoid Research by Agency: FY 1979
(real dollars in thousands)

	Grants		Contracts[a]		Intramural		Total	
	No.	Funds	No.	Funds	No.	Funds	No.	Funds
ADAMHA								
NIDA	54	2,608	10	925	1	3	65	3,536
NIMH	4	145	--	--	3	62	7	207
NIAAA	6	122	--	--	--	--	6	122
NIH								
NCI	2	85	--	--	--	--	2	85
NEI	1	36	--	--	--	--	1	36
NICHD	1	15	--	--	--	--	1	15
NIRR	--	--	--	--	--	--	--	--
NIGMS	1	9	--	--	--	--	1	9
OTHER AGENCIES								
VA	--	--	--	--	8	25	8	25
DOT	--	--	2	104	--	--	2	104
USDA	--	--	1	85	--	--	1	85
TOTAL	69	3,020	13	1,114	12	90	94	4,224

[a]FY '80: RFP 12
 FY '81: RFP 14

Source: Adapted from information provided by NIDA.

investigator-initiated extramural research grants, and most of the rest to extramural contracts. There is relatively little intramural research. The fraction of NIDA grants approved is about 60 percent, but the fraction funded is slightly more than half of that. The total number of cannabis research grants is declining steadily as support (in constant dollars) continues to fall and the average cost of a project (in constant dollars) goes up.

The committee believes that the magnitude of the problem, and the extent and depth of public concern about the consequences of marijuana use warrant more support of research in this field.

TABLE 12   Drug Abuse Research Grant Award Rates and Priority Scores

	1979 Actual	1980 Actual	1981 Estimate	1982 Estimate
Applicants received (number)	359	369	382	360
Percent recommended for approval	59	62	63	62
Percent funded of those approved during year	63	57	40	27
Percent funded of all applicants	37	35	25	20
90 percent priority score	244	230	190	170

Source: Adapted from information provided by NIDA.

Emphasis should be on studies of human beings and other primates, and investigator-initiated research grants should continue to be the primary vehicle of support.

RECOMMENDATIONS

In view of the demonstrated high potential of risk to human health that has been associated with the use of cannabis, the existing funds allocated to such research are not appropriate. The committee's recommendations to federal agencies regarding support of cannabis-related research are:

• More support of cannabis research is needed. Properly allocated, it could pay large dividends in new knowledge and could help to dispel present ignorance in many critical areas. Without this new information, the present level of public anxiety and controversy over the use of marijuana is not likely to be resolved in the forseeable future. Furthermore, we are not likely to improve our present slow progress in developing information about possible therapeutic uses of cannabis and its analogues without the stimulus of increased research grant support. At the end of each of the chapters, we have pointed out opportunities or problems that are ripe at this time.
• A larger proportion of NIDA resources could justifiably be allocated to cannabis research. Without wishing to minimize the value of any of the other drug research programs now supported by NIDA, we believe that the magnitude and social urgency of the marijuana problem warrant a higher priority for cannabis research

than it has apparently received to date. A drug that is currently used by about a third of all American high school seniors, and daily by about one in eleven, deserves more study than we currently are giving it. No other illicit drug is used as widely by our youth, and yet NIDA spent only 9 percent of its research budget on it in FY '80.

* NIDA would be advised to continue its recent policy of reducing the relative proportion of contracts and emphasizing grants. Although we believe that there is need for federal initiatives in stimulating work in neglected areas of current concern, the bulk of research suport should continue to go to investigator-initiated projects.

* The duration for investigator-initiated research should be lengthened beyond the average 3-year period in order to attract and hold good researchers.

* Other agencies should contribute funds for the production, processing, and distribution of cannabis.

* A scientific advisory group should be formed to assist in providing scientific evidence and guidance to the director of NIDA.

* An increased interagency effort targeted toward specific problems not readily addressed by other approaches is required. These would include, for example, human long-term studies, as well as studies in epidemiology, prevention, and treatment. Funds should be contributed by all agencies.

* Research on human beings and other primates should be encouraged, particularly studies in the young. There is a special need at this time for good epidemiological studies that follow identifiable cohorts of marijuana users over a period of time.

REFERENCES

Hurd, Susan. National Heart, Lung, and Blood Institute. Bethesda, Md. Personal communication, 1981.

Little, Francine. National Cancer Institute, Bethesda, Md. Personal communication, 1981.

Leventhal, Carl. National Institute of Arthritis, Metabolism, and Digestive Diseases, Bethesda, Md. Personal communication, 1981.

Ludford, Jacqueline. National Institute on Drug Abuse, Rockville, MD. Personal communication, 1981.

Petersen, Robert. National Institute on Drug Abuse, Rockville, Md. Personal communication, 1981.

Pollin, W. Statement on Drug Abuse Research before the Subcommittee on Alcoholism and Drug Abuse, Committee on Labor and Human Resources. United States Senate, July 27, 1981.

Snyder, Marvin. National Institute on Drug Abuse, Bethesda, Md. Personal communication, 1981.

Appendix

A

WORK OF THE COMMITTEE

To conduct this study, the Institute of Medicine established a committee of experts drawn from relevant disciplines, including clinical medicine, epidemiology, pharmacology, psychiatry, and toxicology. This steering committee's expertise was augmented by consultants, as well as by many other persons serving as panel members. Six panels, each chaired by a committee member, were formed to carry out a detailed analysis of such special issues as the effects of cannabis use on behavioral and psychosocial development, on reproductive and fetal biology, on cardiovascular and respiratory systems, and to consider neurobiologic, genetic, oncogenic, and cytogenetic issues, and cell biology, including pharmacologic and immunologic aspects. During the early months of the study, the panels met to apportion writing responsibilities, and established the scope and focus of each panel's undertaking. The chronology of the panel meetings follows.

February 3, 1981: Panel on Behavioral and Psychosocial Issues met in Washington

February 18, 1981: Panel on Neurobiological Issues met in Washington

February 26, 1981: Panel on Cardiovascular and Respiratory Issues met in New York City

February 27, 1981: Panel on Genetic/Oncogenic/Cytogenetic Issues met in Washington

March 11, 1981: Panel on Reproductive and Fetal Issues met in Boston

March 16, 1981: Subpanel on Intrapersonal Variables and Social Behavior of the Panel on Behavioral and Psychosocial Issues met in Los Angeles

March 23, 1981: Panel on Cell Biology/Pharmacological and Immunological Issues met in Boston

April 14, 1981: Panel on Behavioral and Psychosocial Issues met in Washington

The steering committee, in the meantime, nominated additional candidates for membership on the panels and committee at its first meeting on December 1, 1980. Subsequently, four more meetings were

169

held, on April 15, 1981, June 2-3, 1981, August 31-September 1, 1981, and October 26, 1981. The first two were held in Washington, the third meeting was held in Woods Hole, Massachusetts, and the final meeting was held in Washington.

The committee made full use of research in other countries as well as the United States. A special effort was made to coordinate activities with the staff of the Addiction Research Foundation/World Health Organization Conference on Adverse Health and Behavioral Consequences of Cannabis Use. The group's draft report and working papers were made available to the IOM committee. The mandate of this group was to consider the scientific, clinical, and epidemiological information about potential and actual hazards to health.

Because of widespread public interest in the IOM study, a notice was placed in the February 24, 1981, Federal Register to solicit information from the public and from professional groups on the health-related effects of cannabis use. Approximately 90 responses were received from professional organizations, lawyers, medical doctors, scientists, other professionals, and parents. The responses can be divided into three categories:

1. The dangers of marijuana. The majority of responses came from people and groups opposed to cannabis use. Many parents of cannabis smokers (and ex-cannabis smokers) submitted statements about their personal experiences and observations. Included among the groups that responded are the National Federation of Parents for Drug Free Youth, Georgia Congress of Parents and Teachers, the American Lung Association, Drug Information Program of the Crusade Against Crime, the Committees of Correspondence, Phoenix House Foundation, and Pride.

2. The therapeutic potential of marijuana. Responses were received from medical doctors, as well as individuals or their parents, reporting that cannabis had alleviated pain from various medical problems--rheumatoid arthritis, migraine headaches, multiple sclerosis--and had in some cases lessened the side-effects of drugs used in chemotherapy. In most cases the marijuana had to be obtained by unauthorized means, making many of the victims and their families uncomfortable. Several respondents were from the State of Michigan, where a cannabis therapeutic research program has recently been authorized by the state legislature. Responses were also received from the Alliance for Cannabis Therapeutics and the American Medical Association.

3. Support of general use and legalization of marijuana. Responses in this regard were received from lawyers and other individuals, as well as the following organizations: the Ethiopian Zion Coptic Church, the Cannabis Institute of America, the National Organization for the Reform of Marijuana Laws, and the publication High Times. One writer contended that perhaps more people would submit statements if their anonymity were assured.

Appendix

B

ACCESS TO Δ-9-THC AND MARIJUANA
FOR RESEARCH AND TREATMENT

The investigational use in human subjects of Δ-9-THC and marijuana are controlled by the Federal Food, Drug, and Cosmetic Act and the Investigational New Drug Regulations issued under that Act. In addition, Δ-9-THC and marijuana are controlled under the provisions of the Controlled Substances Act and currently are controlled in Schedule I of the Controlled Substances Act. Schedule I drugs are those that have: (1) high potential for abuse, (2) no currently accepted medical use in treatment in the United States, and (3) lack of accepted safety for use under medical supervision.

Basically two agencies work together for enforcing the controls of the Act: the Food and Drug Administration (FDA) in the Department of Health and Human Services and the Drug Enforcement Administration (DEA) in the Department of Justice. The Department of Justice was petitioned to reconsider the rescheduling of Δ-9-THC and marijuana in 1972, but to date there has been no change. However, DEA and FDA are now under court order to reconsider this situation. An FDA advisory meeting, held in June 1981, considered the scheduling status of the Δ-9-THC capsule only (<u>Federal Register</u>, 1981). The committee recommended that the Δ-9-THC capsule be changed from Schedule I to Schedule II status when a new drug application for Δ-9-THC is approved by FDA. Schedule II drugs are those that have: (1) a high potential for abuse, (2) a currently accepted medical use in treatment in the United States or a currently accepted medical use with severe restrictions, and (3) abuse that may lead to severe psychological or physical dependence.

Complaints and concerns were expressed to the study committee about the supply and distribution of marijuana and Δ-9-THC for treating chemotherapy side-effects in cancer patients. On the one hand, physicians said that there was poor cooperation from federal agencies engaged in controlling and supplying the drug (Koller, 1981; Monsma, 1981), particularly with respect to (1) potency of Δ-9-THC received (concentrations were too low to be effective), and (2) uncertainty and irregularity of the shipments of the drug. On the other hand, some clinicians felt that it was premature to release Δ-9-THC for use in cancer patients (Moertel, 1981; Cook, 1981) because:

* specific indications have not been established, in that the way in which chemotherapeutic agents cause nausea and vomiting is not known;
    * specific populations of patients have not been established;
    * effective dose schedules have not been established;
    * safety of treatment at doses effective for antiemetic purposes remains in question;
    * reported peer-reviewed experience is contradictory and still fragmentary; and
    * controlled, randomized, prospective studies have not been conducted.

Depending upon the use of the drug, two different agencies are in charge of supplying marijuana cigarettes and Δ-9-THC capsules; the National Institute on Drug Abuse (NIDA) controls the supply of marijuana cigarettes and/or Δ-9-THC capsules for basic research, and the National Cancer Institute (NCI) controls the supply of Δ-9-THC capsules for cancer treatment. The processes of obtaining supplies from each agency (or for each purpose) differ.

OBTAINING THE MARIJUANA CIGARETTES*

To obtain marijuana cigarettes for basic research,[†] an investigator must register with DEA (apply for a license), file a Notice of Claimed Investigation Exemption for a New Drug (IND)[††] with FDA, and submit an order for drug substance to NIDA. The agencies suggest that all the paperwork be filed concurrently in order not to unnecessarily delay the process. FDA analyzes the scientific protocol and determines if the project has scientific merit, if the researcher is qualified, and if IND requirements are satisfied. DEA sends an agent to supply the order forms, to determine from local police records whether the investigator has a drug trafficking record, and to see if the investigator has provisions for keeping the drug secure from theft. On notification of approval by FDA and DEA, NIDA will supply the drug. The entire process is supposed to take from 30 days to 6 months, including the visit from the DEA (Tocus, 1981). However, some investigators have contended it can take longer.

To obtain marijuana cigarettes (or Δ-9-THC capsules) for investigational treatment of glaucoma, multiple sclerosis, or

---

*Concentrations of Δ-9-THC range between 0.5 and 2.8 percent; the marijuana cigarettes contain other cannabinoids, as well as other chemicals.

[†]DEA and FDA do not fund research. Federal agencies that have supported cannabis research in FY 1979 (in order of percent cannabinoid research) are: NIDA (84), NIMH (5), NIAA (3), NCI (2), DOT (2), USDA (2), NEI (1), NICHG and NIGMS (less than 1).

[††]Twelve states hold their own IND as of September 1981.

anorexia, the physician must go through the basic research route. In view of the possible contaminant problems with <u>aspergillus</u> and <u>salmonella</u>, it may be necessary to provide sterilized marijuana cigarettes to patients.

OBTAINING THE Δ-9-THC CAPSULES*

As a Schedule I drug, Δ-9-THC can only be used for investigational purposes. However, some cancer patients undergoing chemotherapy treatment and resistant to standard antiemetic drugs benefit from the antiemetic properties of Δ-9-THC. Therefore, a system has been established for the distribution of Δ-9-THC capsules to chemotherapy patients within the guidelines of the Schedule I restrictions.

A physician who wants to dispense Δ-9-THC capsules to his cancer patients does so under NCI Group C distribution system (Group C Guidelines, 1980). The physician sends an FDA registration form to a DEA-approved hospital pharmacy. The pharmacy forwards the application to NCI, which holds its own IND. NCI evaluates the credentials of the physician, and, if approving, informs the pharmacy to supply the physician. This process, under emergency situations, can take as little as 24 hours (Abraham, 1981). A physician may also obtain marijuana cigarettes for cancer patients in an NCI-approved treatment program. More than 500 hospitals have been invited to participate (Abraham, 1981), and about 300 have clearance from DEA (Gunby, 1981). Shipments began late last fall (Gunby, 1981). More than 1,500 physicians have applied, and 1,000 have been approved by DEA (Gunby, 1981). The doses available in capsule form are 2.5 and 5 mg.

At least one company has submitted a New Drug Application (NDA) to the FDA for manufacture of a synthetic Δ-9-THC capsule to treat cancer patients (<u>Federal Register</u>, 1981; Tocus, 1981). If an NDA for Δ-9-THC is approved, a Schedule I status will no longer be appropriate. In fact, the Drug Abuse Advisory Committee[†] recommended that the Δ-9-THC capsule be changed from Schedule I to a Schedule II status when an NDA is approved by FDA.

---

*Purity of Δ-9-THC capsules is better than 96 percent (97-98 percent, C. Turner, 1981, and 100 percent, D. Abraham, 1981).
[†]The committee advises the Commissioner of Food and Drugs regarding the scientific and medical evaluation of all information gathered by the Department of Health and Human Services and the Department of Justice with regard to safety, efficacy, and abuse potential of drugs and other substances and recommends action to be taken by the Department of Health and Human Services with regard to the marketing, investigation, and control of such drugs or other substances.

SUPPLIERS OF MARIJUANA CIGARETTES AND Δ-9-THC CAPSULES

Marijuana cigarettes are supplied to NIDA by Research Triangle Institute, which stores and distributes them (Davignon, 1981).

Many contractors are engaged in the synthesis, storage, and distribution of Δ-9-THC capsules to NCI. Manufacture is done by Aerojet Propulsion Labs (large scale) and Arthur D. Little (small scale). Stanford Research Institute assays Δ-9-THC. Banner Gelatin encapsulates it. Flow Laboratories stores and ships Δ-9-THC to DEA-approved hospital pharmacies.

REFERENCES

Abraham, David. Investigational Drug Branch, Health Science Administration, National Cancer Institute, Bethesda, Md. Personal communication, 1981.

Cook, D.A. Private practice, Bay City, Mich. Personal communication, 1981.

Davignon, Paul. Chief, Pharmaceutical Resources Branch, National Cancer Institute, Bethesda, Md. Personal communication, 1981.

Federal Register, Volume 46, Number 31, February 24, 1981. Study of the health-related effects of marijuana use, pp. 13816-13818, 1981.

Group C Guidelines for the use of Δ-9-Tetrahydrocannabinol NSC134454 for nausea and vomiting induced by antineoplastic chemotherapy. Investigational Drug Branch, Cancer Therapy Evaluation Program, Division of Cancer Treatment, National Cancer Institute, Bethesda, Md., September, 1980.

Gunby, P. Many cancer patients receiving THC as antiemetic. JAMA 245:1515-1518, 1981.

Koller, C.A. Assistant Professor of Internal Medicine, Division of Hematology and Oncology. University of Michigan, Ann Arbor, Mich. Personal communication, 1981.

Moertel, C.G. Director, Mayo Comprehensive Cancer Center; Professor of Oncology, Mayo Medical School; Chairman, Department of Oncology, Mayo Clinic, Rochester, Minn. Personal communication, 1981.

Monsma, Stephen V. Senator, State Senate of Michigan, Lansing, Mich. Personal communication, 1981.

Tocus, Edward C. Chief, Drug Abuse Staff, Food and Drug Administration, Rockville, Md. Personal communication, 1981.

Turner, Carleton. Director, Research Institute of Pharmaceutical Sciences, University of Mississippi, Oxford, Miss. Personal communication, 1981.

C

LONGITUDINAL STUDIES

Appendix C is a review of prospective longitudinal studies of drug use in normal populations listed by completion status, type of sample (school sample, community sample), age of respondents, and year of first contact. Some of the studies are ongoing.

176

Characteristics of Longitudinal Studies of Drug Use in Normal Populations Listed by Completion
Status, Type of Sample, Age of Respondents, and Year of First Contact.

Part 1. Completed Studies: School Samples

Principal Investigators	Population Characteristics	Grade/Age at T1 of Sample Eligible for Panel	Year of First Contact	Year of Last Contact	Total Number of Contacts	Interval Between Contacts	Size of Sample T1 Eligible for Panel	Size of Matched Panel	Methods of Data Collection[a]	Drugs Inquired About
Kellam	All entering public and parochial school first-grade children in a black community in Chicago with low income and high unemployment	Grade 1	1966	1975–1976	5	3 times during first grade 2 years 7 years	1,241	705	Home interviews; school tests (IQ, achievement) and grades; ratings by teacher, clinician, mother (T1–T5); police records, questionnaires (T5)	Cigarettes, beer or wine, hard liquor, marijuana, LSD, other psychedelics, uppers, downers, tranquilizers, cocaine, heroin and other opiates, glue, cough syrup
Smith	Students from grades 4-12 in 6 school systems in greater Boston area, predominantly white and middle-class	Grades 4-11	1969	1973	2-5	1 year	12,000 (approx.)	Variable	Self-administered questionnaires in classrooms; school records; peers' ratings of students' personalities	Cigarettes, liquor, marijuana, ups, downs, psychedelics opiates, inhalants, nonprescription drug store products
Kaplan	Seventh grade students from 18 of 36 junior high schools of the Houston Independent School District	Grade 7	1971	1973	3	1 year	7,620	3,148	Self-administered questionnaires in classrooms	Beer or wine, liquor, marijuana, narcotics
Jessor and Jessor	High school study: random sample of students from grades 7-12 of 3 junior and 3 senior high schools in a small city in the Rocky Mountains, almost all of Anglo-American, middle-class background	Grades 7-9	1969	1972	4	1 year	589	483	Self-administered questionnaires outside of class, school records	Beer or wine, hard liquor, marijuana, amphetamines, LSD, other psychedelics, cocaine, and heroin
		Grades 10-11	1969	1972	2-3	1 year	262	Variable		
Elinson and Josephson	Students from 5 junior and 18 senior high schools purposefully selected to represent varied regions, community sizes, socioeconomic levels, and racial compositions but not to represent the United States	Grades 7-10	1971	1973	2	2 years	18,363	8,136	Self-administered questionnaires in classrooms	Cigarettes, beer or wine, hard liquor, marijuana or hashish, amphetamines, methedrine, barbiturates, LSD, other psychedelics, cocaine, heroin, inhalants

Author	Sample	Grade/Level	Year 1	Year 2	Waves	Duration	N	N	Method	Substances
Annis and Watson	Students of 3 public high schools in a northern Ontario city and dropouts from same classes	Grade 9	(Not Given)	(Not Given)	2	13 months	915	886	Self-administered questionnaires in class; interviews with dropouts at T2	Alcohol, marijuana, tobacco, solvents, hallucinogens, barbiturates, opiates
Kandel	(1) Multistage random sample of New York State public secondary school students from 18 schools and data from mothers or fathers; best school friend in subsample of 5 schools	Grades 9-12	1971	1972	2	6 months	8,206	5,423	Self-administered questionnaires in classrooms (adolescents). Mailed questionnaires (parents)	Cigarettes, beer or wine, hard liquor, marijuana, hashish, amphetamines, methedrine, barbiturates, tranquilizers, LSD, other psychedelics, cocaine, heroin, other narcotics, inhalants, cough syrup
	(2) 1972 Senior class (Third wave)	Grade 12	1971	1973	3	7-12 months	2,386	1,635	Self-administered questionnaires (T1, T2); mailed questionnaires (T3)	Same
Johnston	Youth in Transition cohort--A national random sample of boys in 87 public high schools in continental United States in 1966; drug components added in 1970 and 1974	Grade 10	1966	1974	5	2 years 1 year 1 year 4 years	2,213	1,608	Interviews (T1, T2,T4); self-administered questionnaires (T1-T4); mailed questionnaires (T5); ability tests (T1)	Cigarettes, beer, wine, hard liquor marijuana, amphetamines, barbiturates, hallucinogens, methaqualone, cocaine, heroin
Britt and Campbell	North Carolina high school seniors who expressed an intention to attend college in fall	Grade 12	1961	1962	2	1 year	2,300	1,420	Self-administered questionnaires, (unclear whether in or out of class)	Alcohol
Gulas and King	Seniors at Dartmouth College matched retrospectively to their freshman-year records	College freshmen	Not Given (prior to 1976)	Not Given	2	4 years	90	90	Mailed questionnaires	Marijuana, amphetamines, barbiturates, hallucinogens
Haagen	College juniors at Wesleyan University matched retrospectively to their freshman-and-sophomore-year records	College freshmen	1965	1968	2	3 years	70	70	Self-administered questionnaires; test data on file at Office of Psychological Service	Tobacco, alcohol, marijuana, hallucinogens
Garfield and Garfield	Random sample at large private suburban residential western university	College students	1966-1967	1970-1971	4	1 year	300	T2-100 T3-201 T4-100	Personally administered questionnaires	Alcohol, marijuana, hashish, LSD, mescaline

aThe same methods were used in all waves of data collection of a study, unless specific times are indicated.

Characteristics of Longitudinal Studies of Drug Use in Normal Populations Listed by Completion Status, Type of Sample, Age of Respondents, and Year of First Contact.

Part 1. Completed Studies: School Samples

Principal Investigators	Population Characteristics	Grade/Age at T1 of Sample Eligible for Panel	Year of First Contact	Year of Last Contact	Total Number of Contacts	Interval Between Contacts	Size of Sample T1 Eligible for Panel	Size of Matched Panel	Methods of Data Collection	Drugs Inquired About
Grupp	Random sample of 1% of students at Illinois State University not reporting marijuana use	College undergraduates and graduate students	1969	1973	3	2 years	127	T2-120 T3-103	Personal interviews at T1, T2; mailed questionnaires for those out of area at T2, and for everyone at T3	Marijuana
Goldstein	Students enrolled at Carnegie-Mellon University (class of 1972)	College freshmen	1968	1972	4	Approx: 9 months 16 months 20 months	770	417	Self-administered questionnaires, outside of class (mail technique preserving anonymity)	Beer, hard liquor, marijuana (incl. hashish), tranquilizers and barbiturates, amphetamines, hallucinogens, narcotics, tobacco
Groves	Full-time students at predominantly white nonspecialized colleges with projected enrollment of over 1,000 (1970)	College freshmen and juniors	1970	1971	2	1 year	7,948	3,961	Mailed questionnaires	Caffeine, alcohol, marijuana, hashish methedrine, other amphetamines, barbiturates, sedatives, tranquilizers, LSD, other psychedelics, cocaine, opium, heroin, other narcotics, cough syrups
Mellinger	(1) Probability sample of male freshmen of University of California at Berkeley in Fall 1970	College freshmen	1970	1973	2	2 1/2 years	960	834	Personal interviews and self-administered forms; school records; mailed questionnaires	Tobacco, alcohol, marijuana or hashish, amphetamines, barbiturates, sedatives, psychedelics, cocaine, heroin, opium, other opiates, inhalants
	(2) Probability sample of senior men in class of 1971	College seniors	1971	1973	2	2 1/2 years	986	821	Same	Same
Jessor and Jessor	College study--random sample of arts and science university students in a small Rocky Mountain city	College freshmen	1970	1973	4	1 year	276	226	Self-administered questionnaires; school records	Beer or wine, hard liquor, marijuana, amphetamines, LSD, other psychedelics, cocaine, heroin

Author	Sample	Subject	Year start	Year end	Times	Interval	N (initial)	N (final)	Method	Drugs
Schuckit	Random samples of incoming freshmen at:									
	(1) Washington University in St. Louis	College freshmen	1970	1974	4	1 year	158	Not Given	Semistructured interviews: mailed questionnaires to nonresidents	Tobacco, alcohol, marijuana, hashish, amphetamines, speed, LSD, mescaline, psilocybin, STP, MDA, opiates, medicinal drugs
	(2) University of California at San Diego	College freshmen	1971	1975	4	1 year	222	188		
Ginsberg and Greenley	Students enrolled at University of Wisconsin-Madison 1971-1974	College freshmen and sophomores	1971	1974	2	2 years	319	274	Mailed questionnaires	Marijuana
Sadava	(1) College freshmen in an English-language Roman Catholic college in province of Quebec	College freshmen	Not Given (prior to 1973)	Not Given	2	6 months	358	319	Self-administered questionnaires in classrooms	Cannabis, psychedelics, amphetamines, alcohol
	(2) Undergraduates at a small Ontario university in introductory psychology course	College freshmen and sophomores	1972	1973	2	6 months	467	374	Self-administered questionnaires	Alcohol, tobacco, marijuana and other illicit drugs
Kay	Random sample of male students entering Lehigh University	College freshmen	1971 1972 1973	1974 1974 1974	4 3 2	6 months: 1-T2; 1 year; T2-T3, T3-T4	130 124 112	68 85 98	Self-administered questionnaires, adjective check list, California Psychological Inventory	Marijuana
Moos	Entering classes of two universities	College freshmen	Not Given	Not Given	3	9 months 3 years	1,296	T2-886 T3-567	Self-administered questionnaires, outside class	Alcohol

Characteristics of Longitudinal Studies of Drug Use in Normal Populations Listed by Completion Status, Type of Sample, Age of Respondents, and Year of First Contact.

Part 2. Completed Studies: Community Samples

Principal Investigators	Population Characteristics	Grade/Age at T1 of Sample Eligible for Panel	Year of First Contact	Year of Last Contact	Total Number of Contacts	Interval Between Contacts	Size of Sample T1 Eligible for Panel	Size of Matched Panel	Methods of Data Collection	Drugs Inquired About
Lukoff and Brook	Samples of ghetto community stratified for ethnicity, social class, and contiguity with deviance:									
	(1) Children	13-17 yrs	1973	1975-1976	2	3 years	403	183	Household interviews	Marijuana, ups, downs, psychedelics, heroin
	(2) Mothers	30-45 yrs					284	183		
Brunswick	Representative community sample of Harlem youth	16-17 years old	1969-1970	1975-1976	2	6 years	664	536	Household interviews	Alcohol, marijuana, amphetamines, barbiturates, acid, cocaine, heroin, glue
Sieber	19 year old conscripts born in canton of Zurich who report some alcohol/drug use at initial contact	19 years	1971	1974	2	3 years	1,413	841	Self-administered questionnaires T1; mailed questionnaires T2	Alcohol, tobacco, marijuana
Robins	(1) Vietnam veterans random sample of army enlisted males who returned from Vietnam to the United States in September 1971, and a supplementary random sample from all men returning that month whose urine had been detected as positive for morphine prior to leaving Vietnam. T2 sampled from reduced T1 target population restricted to men inducted since 1969 and from the 25 more populous states	20 years (mean)	1972	1974 1975	2	2 years	605	571	Interviews; urine samples; military and Veterans' Administration records	Cigarettes, alcohol, marijuana, amphetamines, barbiturates, tranquilizers, hallucinogens, cocaine, narcotics

181

Study	Sample	Age	Years (T1)	Year (T2)	Waves	Interval	N (T1)	N (T2)	Method	Variables
	(2) Control group at T2--sample of non-veterans matched on Selective Service Board, draft eligibility, age, and education	Matched to veterans	1974-1975	--	1	--	302	284	Interviews; urine samples; Selective Service Records	Same
Cahalan et al.	(1) National probability sample of United States adult population; (T2) sampled from reduced T1 target population N=1,810, with abstainers and very infrequent drinkers subsampled at a lesser rate	21 and over	1964-1965	1967	2	2 years	1,810	1,359	Household interviews (T1); mail questionnaires	Drinking patterns, practices, and problems
	(2) National probability sample of white males aged 21-59, with oversampling of urban areas	21-59 years old	1969	1973	2	4 years	978	725	Same	Same
	(3) Probability sample of white males, aged 21-59, in San Francisco	21-59 years old	1967-1968	1972	2	4 years	786	615	Same	Same

Characteristics of Longitudinal Studies of Drug Use in Normal Populations Listed by Completion Status, Type of Sample, Age of Respondents, and Year of First Contact.

Part 3. Ongoing Studies: A—Within Adolescence, Adulthood

Principal Investigators	Population Characteristics	Grade/Age at T1 of Sample Eligible for Panel	Year of First Contact	Year of Last Contact	Total Number of Contacts	Interval Between Contacts	Size of Sample T1 Eligible for Panel	Size of Matched Panel	Methods of Data Collection	Drugs Inquired About
Huba and Bentler	Students in the greater Los Angeles area with oversampling of lower socio-economic schools	Grades 7-9	1976	1980[a]	4	1 year 2 years 1 year	1,634	768	Self-administered questionnaires from the students, parents (T1,T4) and peers (T1,T2)	Cigarettes, beer, wine, liquor, marijuana, hashish, coffee, minor and major tranquilizers, barbiturates, sedatives, antidepressants, amphetamines, non-amphetamines, uppers, LSD, other psychedelics, sniffing stuff, amyl nitrate, nonprescription: sleeping pills, stimulants, cough medicine, cold medicine, cocaine, heroin, other narcotics, PCP, coca paste
Lukoff and Brook	Quota sample from 6 states (Connecticut, Kansas, New Jersey, New York, Ohio, and South Carolina). Approximately equal numbers of males and females, blacks and whites of middle socioeconomic status	Grades 9-10	1979	1981	2	2 years	932	Not yet completed	Self administered questionnaires	Alcohol, cigarettes, marijuana, amphetamines, barbiturates, LSD, other psychedelics, heroin, other narcotics, tranquilizers, quaaludes, cocaine, inhalants
Clayton and Voss	Nationally representative sample of men born between 1944 and 1954 inclusive, who registered with Selective Service upon age 18	20-30 years old	1974-1975	1982	2	6-7 years	450	Not yet completed	Personal interviews	Cigarettes, alcohol, marijuana, psychedelics, stimulants, sedatives, heroin, other opiates, cocaine, tranquilizers, inhalants

Part 3. Ongoing Studies: B--From Adolescence to Young Adulthood

Investigators	Sample	Age/Grade	Year started	Latest	No. contacts	Interval	Sample size	Completion	Methods	Substances
Carpenter, Lester, Pandina, and Labouvie	Cohort-sequential design--Random samples of New Jersey adolescents-- a) 9 cohorts born 1967-75 b) 3 cohorts born 1964-66 c) 3 cohorts born 1961-63 d) 3 control groups at T4	a) 12 years b) 15 years c) 18 years	1979	ongoing	14 telephone 8 onsite	1 year 3 years until age 24; 6 years after age 24	a)1,350 b) 450 c) 450 d) 150	Not yet completed	On-site: -personal interviews -self-administered questionnaires -behavioral tests -blood sample -psychological test -medical exams Telephone contact: -major life events -alcohol and drug taking outcomes	Alcohol, cigarettes, marijuana, amphetamines, barbiturates, LSD, other psychedelics, heroin, other narcotics, tranquilizers, quaaludes, cocaine, inhalants, PCP, amyl and butyl nitrates, over-the-counter psychotherapeutics, caffeine
Elliott	National Youth Survey-National probability multistage cluster sample of dwellings	11-17 years	1976	1980	5	1 year	1,725	T2-1655 T3-1626 T4-1543 T5-1494	Personal structured interviews	Tobacco, beer, wine, liquor, marijuana, hallucinogens, cocaine, heroin, medical and non-medical use of amphetamines, barbiturates
Jessor, Jessor, and Donovan	Young adult follow-up. High school sample--random sample of students from grades 7-9 of 3 junior high schools in a small city in the Rocky Mountains, almost all of Anglo-American, middle class background	Grades 7-9	1969	1981[a]	6	1 year 1 year 1 year 7 years 2 years	432	Not yet completed	T1-T4--Self-administered questionnaires in school (high school sample) in small groups (college sample)	Beer, wine, hard liquor, marijuana, LSD, amphetamines, cocaine, heroin, tranquilizers, barbiturates, morphine
	College sample--random sample of freshman class arts and science university students in a small Rocky Mountain city	College freshman	1970	1981[a]	6	1 year 1 year 1 year 6 years 2 years	205	not yet completed	T5,T6--Adult follow-ups: mailed self-administered questionnaires	

[a]Future contacts planned, if funds available.

Characteristics of Longitudinal Studies of Drug Use in Normal Populations Listed by Completion Status, Type of Sample, Age of Respondents, and Year of First Contact.

Part 3. Ongoing Studies: B--From Adolescence to Young Adulthood

Principal Investigators	Population Characteristics	Grade/Age at T1 of Sample Eligible for Panel	Year of First Contact	Year of Last Contact	Total Number of Contacts	Interval Between Contacts	Size of Sample T1 Eligible for Panel	Size of Matched Panel	Methods of Data Collection	Drugs Inquired About
Johnston and Bachman	Monitoring the Future--cohort sequential design. Successive nationally representative cohorts of high school seniors from 115 public and 15 private high schools; repeated annually; entire senior classes in schools with 300 seniors, and subsamples (N=300) in larger schools	Grade 12	1975-ongoing	ongoing	11 for each cohort	1 year for each cohort (2 yrs for each cohort 1/2 sample)	2,400 (target for each cohort; 1,200 for each cohort 1/2 sample)	Not yet completed	T1--Self-administered questionnaires in classrooms T2, adult follow-ups -- Mailed questionnaires	Alcohol, cigarettes, marijuana, amphetamines, barbiturates, LSD, other psychedelics, heroin, other narcotics, tranquilizers, quaaludes, cocaine, inhalants, PCP, amyl and butyl nitrates, over-the-counter psychotherapeutics, caffeine
Kandel	Multistage random sample of adolescents enrolled in New York public secondary school selected from 18 schools a) regular students b) absentees	Grades 10-11	1971	1980[a]	3	6 months 9 years	a) 1,321 b) 330	1,081 244	T1,T2--Self-administered questionnaires in classrooms T3--Adult follow-up--Household interviews	Cigarettes, beer or wine, hard liquor, marijuana, hashish, methedrine, LSD, other psychedelics, cocaine, heroin, other narcotics, inhalants, cough syrup, stimulants, sedatives and tranquilizers (medical and non-medical use)

	Sample								Method	Substances
Kaplan	Seventh grade students enrolled in 18 of 36 junior high schools of the Houston Independent School District	1971	1981–1982	Grade 7	4	1 year / 1 year / 9–11 years	9,300	Not yet completed	T1–T3—Self-administered questionnaires; T4—Adult follow-up—Household interviews	Marijuana/hashish, barbiturates, inhalants, hallucinogens, amphetamines, tranquilizers, heroin, other narcotics, quaaludes, cocaine
Lauer and Akers	All students in 2 junior high schools, 1 senior high school in small Iowa city	1980	1984	7–12	5	1 year	2,194	Not yet completed	Self-administered questionnaires in classroom; Saliva test	Cigarettes, chewing tobacco, snuff, cigars/pipe
Schlegel	Random sample of students in 2 school boards (urban, rural) in southern Ontario	1974	1980[a]	9–12	7	4 months / 4 months / 4 months / 1 year / 2 years / 2 years	1,781	918	(T1–T4) Self-administered questionnaires in classroom. (T5–T7) Mailed self-administered questionnaires	Beer, wine, liquor, cigarettes, amphetamines, barbiturates, marijuana, hallucinogens, tranquilizers, heroin, glue
Smith	Students and former students in middle-class predominantly white school district in the greater Boston area	1969	1981	Grades 8–10	4–6	1 year / 1 year / 1 year / 1 year / 8 years	1,935	Not yet completed	T1–T5—Self-administered questionnaires, peer ratings of personality, school records; T6—Adult follow-up - Mailed questionnaires	Cigarettes, beer, wine, liquor, marijuana, hashish, ups, downs, tripping stuff, cocaine, heroin and other opiates, drug store medicine, sniffing stuff, combination drugs

[a]Future contacts planned, if funds available.

Appendix
D

PARAQUAT ISSUE

Paraquat is a herbicide that is used throughout the world. It is available in an aerosol form, granules, and a water-soluble concentrate. As a result of accidental or suicidal swallowing of the water-soluble concentrate, more than 500 human fatalities have occurred (Harley et al., 1977). In contrast, neither inhalation of the spray nor ingestion of paraquat granules has been shown to be of clinical importance (Fairshter and Wilson, 1975).

About 60 percent of the marijuana consumed in the United States is grown in Mexico. Since 1975, in the attempt to reduce the illegal production of marijuana, the Mexican government has been spraying marijuana fields from airplanes. The herbicide kills the treated plants within 1 or 2 days. Marijuana producers have resorted to harvesting the plants soon after spraying, minimizing exposure to sunshine, so that they are not destroyed. The paraquat persists on the dried leaves. Samples of marijuana confiscated at the U.S.-Mexico border have disclosed that about 21 percent of the confiscated marijuana was contaminated with paraquat in varying concentrations.

Paraquat damages the lungs, heart, kidneys, adrenal glands, central nervous system, liver, skeletal muscle, and spleen. In general, all effects but those on the lungs are transitory. The changes in the lungs of humans after ingestion appear to be dose-related: small amounts of the swallowed chemical may cause modest and reversible lung damage; in contrast, larger quantities cause lethal pulmonary fibrosis. An important element in paraquat toxicity is the fact that it is concentrated in the lungs where it does particular damage to the alveolar lining. In many respects, probably including the mechanism by which it damages the lungs, its effects resemble those of oxygen toxicity but seem to be less reversible (Smith and Heath, 1976).

With respect to marijuana, the use of paraquat as a herbicide entails the possibility of risk to two populations: (1) those who spray the paraquat and the workers in the fields who are exposed to an environment containing the paraquat spray, and (2) the marijuana smoker. To date, no toxic effects attributable to paraquat, per se, have been proved in either population. However, the observations thus far relate to the acute hazards of paraquat inhalation and do not provide any assurance about the long-term effects. Indeed, observations on other inhaled toxins suggest that exposure for many years may be prerequisite for the development of clinical disability.

An important question with respect to the toxic effects of paraquat on the lungs is how much of the paraquat survives combustion and is transferred in the smoke to the gas-exchanging surfaces of the lungs. Studies conducted by NIDA indicate that as much as 0.2 percent of the paraquat in a marijuana cigarette appeared in a condensate of smoke prepared under laboratory conditions. The results suggested that a typical marijuana cigarette contaminated at approximately 500 ppm--a reasonable degree of contamination--would produce smoke containing up to 1 mg of paraquat. This experimental evidence has led to the prediction that a human smoker of five marijuana cigarettes per day would expose the lungs to approximately 5 mg of paraquat. Laboratory evidence derived from hamsters suggests the possibility of damaging the distal part of the airways (the bronchioles and the proximal alveolar ducts) by this exposure. These experiments and predictions suggest that an individual who continued to smoke paraquat-contaminated cigarettes would be a candidate for serious lung injury. The prospect probably would be greatly heightened by the toxic effects of the combusted marijuana.

There are only a few observations of experimental animals that bear directly on the effects of inhaled paraquat (Kimbrough and Gaines, 1970; Zavala and Rhodes, 1978). These suggest that similar lesions are produced by ingested paraquat and by paraquat introduced into the airways. For example, the introduction of minute quantities of paraquat dichloride intrabronchially, in concentrations ranging from 10 mg to 100 mg, elicited focal pulmonary edema, hemorrhage, and fibrosis (Zavala and Rhodes, 1978). The smaller doses are within the range to which a smoker of marijuana contaminated by paraquat might be exposed. However, the experimental evidence is not entirely relevant on several accounts: (1) paraquat arriving at the lung surfaces by inhalation from contaminated air or after smoking must be carried in the form of smoke, gas, or small droplets, because larger droplets, such as the aerosols used in agriculture, are apt to precipitate out in proximal airways, which are protected by cilia and mucus; (2) the intrabronchial installation of paraquat in a solution provides a different pattern of access to the gas-exchanging surfaces of the lungs than does inhalation of smoke, gas, or droplets; (3) because of its water solubility, paraquat that escapes pyrolyzation during smoking would be expected to be taken up by the tracheal bronchial tree and its branches before reaching the alveoli unless carried in the form of smoke, gas, or small droplets.

In essence, the evidence concerning the injurious effects of paraquat inhaled after either spraying or smoking is too meager for conclusions. The observations available since 1975 have not proved that paraquat, per se, is harmful to the lungs. On the other hand, the clinical experience to date, coupled with the increasing understanding of the biochemical basis for paraquat toxicity, raises the serious possibility that continued exposure to inhaled paraquat is likely to be harmful to the lungs, that the predominant effect will be diffuse interstitial fibrosis, and that if exposure is sufficiently intense over years, respiratory insufficiency, disability, and death may reasonably be expected to ensue.

REFERENCES

Fairshter, R.D. and Wilson, A.F. Paraquat poisoning: Manifestations and therapy. Am. J. Med. 59:751-753, 1975.

Harley, J.B., Grinspan, S., and Root, R.K. Paraquat suicide in a young woman: Results of therapy directed against the superoxide radical. Yale J. Biol. Med. 50:481-488, 1977.

Kimbrough, R.D. and Gaines, T.B. Toxicity of paraquat to rats and its effect on rat lungs. Toxicol. Appl. Pharmacol. 17:679-690, 1970.

Smith, P. and Heath, D. Paraquat. CRC Crit. Rev. Toxicol. 4:411-445, 1976.

Zavala, D.C. and Rhodes, M.L. An effect of paraquat on the lungs of rabbits. Chest 74:418-420, 1978.